全国高等医药院校精品教材

Bilingual Fundamental Nursing Skill Training Guide

基础护理学双语实验指导

主　审　李曾艳
主　编　杜　玲
编　者　(以姓氏笔画为序)
王姝力　刘　妍　那　娜
张　颖　张冠如　杜　玲
姚　婕　宫丽曼

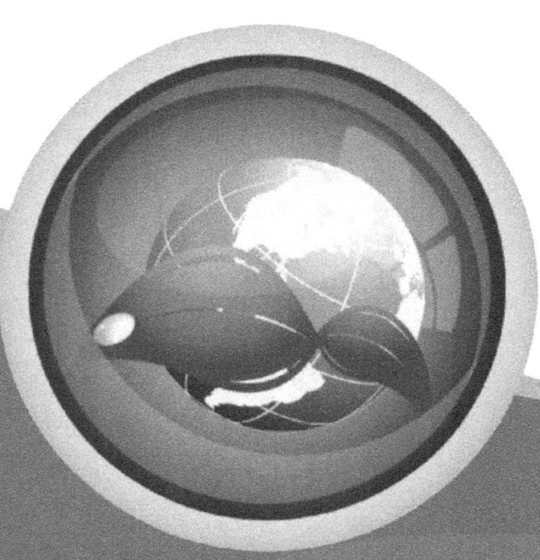

華中科技大學出版社
http://www.hustp.com
中国·武汉

内 容 简 介

本教材采用双语编写，主要内容为护理学专业基本操作技术，采用中英文对照的形式阐述护理学操作目的、评估、物品准备、操作过程、护理事项、沟通模板、评分细则等内容。将护理专业英语与操作技能有机结合。各项操作内容均按照临床一线最新操作标准编著，新增英文的沟通模板可以为涉外护理人员提供良好的沟通素材，附录中补充的护理交接班模板可以为学生提供参考。

图书在版编目(CIP)数据

基础护理学双语实验指导/杜玲主编. —武汉：华中科技大学出版社，2013.8
ISBN 978-7-5609-9355-3

Ⅰ.基… Ⅱ.杜… Ⅲ.护理学-双语教学-教学参考资料 Ⅳ.R47

中国版本图书馆 CIP 数据核字(2013)第 207558 号

基础护理学双语实验指导 杜 玲 主编

策划编辑：居 颖
责任编辑：居 颖 程 芳
封面设计：范翠璇
责任校对：马燕红
责任监印：徐 露
出版发行：华中科技大学出版社(中国·武汉) 电话：(027)81321913
武汉市东湖新技术开发区华工科技园 邮编：430223
录 排：华中科技大学惠友文印中心
印 刷：北京虎彩文化传播有限公司
开 本：787mm×1092mm 1/16
印 张：13
字 数：259 千字
版 次：2019 年 3 月第 1 版第 7 次印刷
定 价：32.00 元

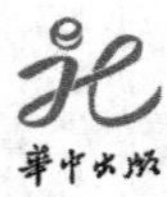

前言

Qianyan

基础护理技术是每名护生必须掌握的基本技能，是护生基础学习阶段和临床实习前需要加强训练的主要内容。随着医学模式的转变和人们健康意识的增强，“以人为中心”的整体护理理念逐渐在工作中得到体现，最大限度地满足服务对象的全方位需求已经成为临床护理的重要课题之一。在护理教学中如何运用护理程序、如何理论联系实际、如何在护理操作中与患者有效沟通、提高学生分析问题和解决问题的能力是教学中的重点。另外，随着我国对外学术交流的不断深入，社会对专业技术人员的外语水平要求也越来越高。为适应当今社会对护理专业人才培养的要求，本教材采用双语编写，主要内容为基础护理学操作目的、评估、物品准备、操作过程、护理事项、沟通模板、评分细则等内容。按照临床一线最新操作要求编写的相关操作可以让学生尽快掌握与临床工作接轨的操作技术，更好地适应临床工作。为方便学生学习，特别在重要词汇下画波浪线进行强调。这是一本能够为师生提供应用性操作标准的双语参考书，旨在为学生提高专业英语的应用能力，更好地适应临床实习打好基础。

本教材虽经编者精心推敲与仔细核对，但纰漏和错误之处仍在所难免，恳请相关专家、学者和热心读者不吝赐教。

编　者

Contents

Chapter 1
Bed-making
铺 床 法

1.1 Making a Closed Bed
铺 备 用 床

Purpose 操作目的

1. To keep the ward neat.
保持病室整洁。
2. To prepare for a newly admitted patient.
准备接收新患者。

Assessment 评估

1. Check whether other patients in the ward are receiving therapy or dining.
检查病室内其他患者是否正在进行治疗或进餐。
2. Assess whether the hospital bed and linens are in good condition, whether the quilt is suitable for the season.
评估患者及床上用物是否完好,被子是否适合季节需要。

Gather equipment 物品准备

Equipments:护理车上(由上至下)依次为 pillow 枕芯,pillowcase 枕套,quilt or

blanket 棉胎或毛毯，quilt cover 被套，large sheet 大单，mattress pad 床褥，hand sanitizer 洗手液，bed brush 床刷，bed brush cover(if necessary)床刷套(按需准备)。

Procedure 操作过程

1. Report and tidy your dress.

报告并整理仪表。

2. Check the validity of hand sanitizer and wash hands in 7 steps and put on the mask.

检查洗手液的有效期，7 步洗手法洗手并戴口罩。

3. Prepare the equipments. Place linens on the nursing trolley in order of use.

准备用物，按使用顺序将用物置于护理车上。

4. Wash hands and remove the mask.

洗手、摘口罩。

5. Take all the equipment to the patient's bedside.

携用物至患者床旁。

6. Assess the environment. Wash hands and put on the mask.

评估环境，洗手、戴口罩。

7. Move the bedside table about 20 cm away from the bed.

移开床旁桌，使其距离床约 20 cm。

8. Move the bedside chair next to the foot of the bed.

将床旁椅移至床尾。

9. Place linens on the chair in order of use. Move the nursing trolley to the middle of the ward.

按使用顺序将床上用物放在椅子上。将护理车置于病室中间。

10. Check the mattress and turn it over as needed. Move it up to the head of the bed and center it.

检查床垫并根据需要翻转床垫。将床垫往上推，居中齐床头。

11. Align the mattress pad flat out on the mattress.

将床褥对齐床头，平铺于床垫上。

12. Place a large sheet on the mattress with its horizontal and vertical center folds at the center lines of the mattress.

将大单放在床垫上，使其横中线和纵中线对齐床垫的相应中线。

13. Unfold the large sheet in sequence from the head to the foot of the bed, from

the near side to the opposite side.

从床头到床尾、从近侧到对侧依次打开大单。

14. Tuck the excess large sheet under the head of the mattress.

将床头余下部分的大单折入床垫下。

15. Make a mitered corner at the head of the bed on the near side.

铺近侧床头角(包角)。

16. Making a mitered corner: Lifts the corner of the mattress with your right hand, and folds the rest part of the large sheet under the mattress with your left hand. Lift the edge of the large sheet 30 cm away from the head of a bed, make the lifting part looks like an equilateral triangle, and then fold two angles under the mattress respectively.

包角:右手托起床垫一角,另一手伸过床头中线将大单折入床垫下,在距离床头约30 cm处,向上提起大单边缘,使大单头端呈等边三角形,再分别将两角塞于床垫下。

17. Move to the foot of the bed, tuck the excess large sheet under the foot of the mattress, make a mitered corner in the same way for the head of the bed on the same side.

移至床尾,将床尾余下部分的大单折入床垫下,同法包好同侧床尾角。

18. Move to the center of the bed, tuck the remainder of the large sheet's center part under the mattress.

移至床中部,将大单中部边缘塞于床垫下。

19. Move to the opposite side of the bed, repeat steps 12-18 to make the large sheet on the opposite side. At last pull the large sheet toward you and straighten out the sheet to make sure that there are no wrinkles in it.

转至床对侧,重复步骤12～18同法铺好对侧大单。最后将大单向一侧牵拉确保床单没有褶皱。

20. Place the quilt cover on the bed with its vertical center fold at the vertical center line of the bed and with the top of the quilt cover placed so that the hem is 15 cm away from the head of the bed.

将被套放在床上,使其纵中线对齐床的纵中线,被套上缘距离床头15 cm。

21. Unfold the quilt cover in sequence, draw its end of upper-layer upwards from its placket.

依次打开被套,将被套尾部开口端上层向上打开1/3处。

22. Place the quilt folded in "S" form into the placket of the quilt cover so that its end is even with the end of the quilt cover.

将“S”形折叠的棉胎放入被套尾端开口处，棉胎底边与被套开口边缘平齐。

23. Pull the top of the quilt into the top of the quilt cover with your left hand.

用左手将棉胎上端拉至被套顶端。

24. Unfold the quilt and make it even with the quilt cover.

展开棉胎，使其平铺于被套内。

25. Unfold the end of the quilt and make it even with the quilt cover in the same way, tie the open end of the quilt cover.

用同样的方法展开棉胎尾部于被套内后拉平被套，系带打结。

26. Tuck in the two side edges of the quilt along the edges of the bed and tuck in its end along the end of the bed.

将盖被两侧平齐床缘内折，尾端平齐床尾内折。

27. Open the pillowcase and slip it over the pillow. Tie the open end of the pillowcase.

打开枕套并套于枕芯外，系带打结。

28. Place the pillow in an upright position at the head of the bed with the open end of the pillowcase facing away from the door of the room.

将枕头横放于床头，枕套开口端背门。

29. Return the bedside table and chair.

移回床旁桌和床旁椅。

30. Wash hands and remove the mask.

洗手、摘口罩。

Nurse Alert 护理事项

1. While making the bed, there should be no patients in the ward receiving therapy or dining.

铺床时，病室内应没有患者进行治疗或进餐。

2. Always use good body mechanics to conserve time and energy. For example, when you place an adjustable bed in the high position and drop the bed side rails, using correct posture can reduce strain on you as you work.

运用人体力学原理以省时和节力。例如，将升降床升起、将床栏放下等动作若采取正确姿势可以减轻操作者的肌肉疲劳。

3. Smooth the bed so that it is free of wrinkles to avoid irritating patient's skin and causing discomfort.

床铺平整无褶皱，以免刺激患者皮肤及引起不适。

New Words and Expressions
单 词 表

quilt [kwilt] *n.* 被子；棉胎

mattress ['mætris] *n.* 床垫；褥子；空气垫

horizontal [hɔri'zɔntəl] *adj.* 水平的；地平线的；同一阶层的

vertical ['və:tikəl] *adj.* 垂直的，直立的；头顶的，顶点的

tuck [tʌk] *vt.* 卷起；挤进；用某物舒适地裹住

wrinkle ['riŋkl] *n.* 皱纹；皱褶

hem [hem] *n.* 边，边缘；摺边

placket ['plækit] *n.* 开口

Communication Model
沟 通 模 板

Self-introduction Model 常规介绍模板

Good morning/afternoon teachers, my name is ××, I come from class ××, my student's number is ××. Today, I am going to show you the process of making a closed bed, the equipments I have prepared are... ,everything is ready, may I start?

老师上午/下午好，我是××，来自××班，我的学号为××。今天我要展示的操作是铺床法，所准备的用物有……，准备完毕，请求开始。

Assessment 评估

There is no patient receiving therapy or dining in the ward. The bed and linens are in good condition and suitable for the season.

病室内无人进餐或治疗。床上用品完好，被服符合季节要求。

Scoring Criteria 1

评分细则 1

<table>
<tr><th colspan="2">项　目</th><th>总分</th><th>技术操作要求</th><th>标准分</th><th>扣分说明</th><th>得分</th></tr>
<tr><td rowspan="4">评估
10</td><td>仪表</td><td>2</td><td>仪表端庄、服装整洁、修剪指甲、洗手戴口罩</td><td>2</td><td>一项不符扣 2 分</td><td></td></tr>
<tr><td rowspan="2">物品</td><td rowspan="2">6</td><td>用物齐备</td><td>4</td><td>一项不符扣 1 分</td><td></td></tr>
<tr><td>治疗车上下放置合理</td><td>2</td><td>一项不符扣 1 分</td><td></td></tr>
<tr><td>环境</td><td>2</td><td>用物按顺序摆放，并能按顺序说出物品</td><td>2</td><td>一项不符扣 1 分</td><td></td></tr>
<tr><td rowspan="26">实施
70</td><td rowspan="4">铺床褥</td><td rowspan="4">12</td><td>移开床旁桌和床旁椅位置得当、动作轻稳</td><td>4</td><td>一项不符扣 1 分</td><td></td></tr>
<tr><td>根据需要翻转床垫</td><td>2</td><td>一项不符扣 2 分</td><td></td></tr>
<tr><td>床褥放置位置方法正确</td><td>2</td><td>一项不符扣 2 分</td><td></td></tr>
<tr><td>床褥展开方法正确、展开平整</td><td>4</td><td>一项不符扣 1 分</td><td></td></tr>
<tr><td rowspan="6">铺大单</td><td rowspan="6">20</td><td>大单放置正确、一次展开</td><td>2</td><td>一项不符扣 1 分</td><td></td></tr>
<tr><td>铺单手法、顺序正确</td><td>4</td><td>一项不符扣 1 分</td><td></td></tr>
<tr><td>折角手法、顺序正确</td><td>4</td><td>一项不符扣 2 分</td><td></td></tr>
<tr><td>中线正</td><td>2</td><td>一项不符扣 2 分</td><td></td></tr>
<tr><td>床角及边缘整齐、紧扎、美观</td><td>6</td><td>一项不符扣 2 分</td><td></td></tr>
<tr><td>床面平整、美观</td><td>2</td><td>一项不符扣 1 分</td><td></td></tr>
<tr><td rowspan="8">套被套</td><td rowspan="8">24</td><td>被套放置合理、一次展开</td><td>2</td><td>一项不符扣 1 分</td><td></td></tr>
<tr><td>棉胎放置合理、展开方法正确</td><td>4</td><td>一项不符扣 2 分</td><td></td></tr>
<tr><td>套棉胎方法正确</td><td>4</td><td>一项不符扣 2 分</td><td></td></tr>
<tr><td>被套两侧对称、齐床沿</td><td>4</td><td>一项不符扣 2 分</td><td></td></tr>
<tr><td>被套中线与床中线齐</td><td>2</td><td>一项不符扣 1 分</td><td></td></tr>
<tr><td>被尾折叠平整、齐床尾，系带无外露</td><td>4</td><td>一项不符扣 2 分</td><td></td></tr>
<tr><td>被头充实，与床头距离适宜(15 cm)</td><td>2</td><td>一项不符扣 1 分</td><td></td></tr>
<tr><td>被套内外平整、美观</td><td>2</td><td>一项不符扣 1 分</td><td></td></tr>
<tr><td rowspan="4">套枕套</td><td rowspan="4">8</td><td>在床尾或椅子上套枕套，方法正确</td><td>2</td><td>一项不符扣 2 分</td><td></td></tr>
<tr><td>枕头四角平整、充实</td><td>2</td><td>一项不符扣 1 分</td><td></td></tr>
<tr><td>枕头摆放方式正确</td><td>2</td><td>一项不符扣 2 分</td><td></td></tr>
<tr><td>枕头放置正确，开口背门</td><td>2</td><td>一项不符扣 1 分</td><td></td></tr>
<tr><td rowspan="2">整理</td><td rowspan="2">6</td><td>移回床旁桌和床旁椅、动作轻稳</td><td>2</td><td>一项不符扣 1 分</td><td></td></tr>
<tr><td>用物处理正确，洗手</td><td>4</td><td>一项不符扣 2 分</td><td></td></tr>
<tr style="display:none"><td></td></tr>
<tr style="display:none"><td></td></tr>
<tr><td rowspan="4">评价
20</td><td rowspan="2">能力</td><td rowspan="2">6</td><td>语言流畅，有效沟通</td><td>3</td><td>一项不符扣 2 分</td><td></td></tr>
<tr><td>按规定时间完成(5 min)</td><td>3</td><td>每超过 30 s 扣 1 分</td><td></td></tr>
<tr><td>英语</td><td>10</td><td>发音准确，语言流畅，关爱患者，符合逻辑</td><td>10</td><td>一项不符扣 2 分</td><td></td></tr>
<tr><td>效果</td><td>4</td><td>床单元整体符合要求，护士操作符合力学原理</td><td>4</td><td>一项不符扣 2 分</td><td></td></tr>
<tr><td colspan="3">主考教师签字：</td><td>日期：</td><td colspan="2">总分：100</td><td>得分：</td></tr>
</table>

评分标准：91～100 分为优，81～90 分为良，71～80 分为中，60～70 分为差，低于 60 分为不及格。

1.2 Making an Unoccupied Bed
铺暂空床

Purpose 操作目的

1. To keep the ward neat.

保持病室整洁。

2. To prepare for the patient who is newly admitted or when the hospitalized patient needs to be off for examination or therapy.

供新入院患者或住院患者暂时离床(如外出检查或治疗)时使用。

Assessment 评估

1. Obtain health information from the patient admitted.

了解新入院患者的病情。

2. Assess the hospitalized patient's health condition, whether he/she is allowed to be up and about or be off for examination or therapy.

评估住院患者的病情,他/她是否被允许暂时离床活动或外出检查治疗。

Gather equipment 物品准备

Equipments:根据需要备 pillowcase 枕套,quilt cover 被套,large sheet 大单,hand sanitizer 洗手液,bed brush 床刷,bed brush cover 床刷套。

Procedure 操作过程

1. Report and tidy your dress.

报告并整理仪表。

2. Check the validity of hand sanitizer and wash hands in 7 steps and put on the mask.

检查洗手液的有效期,7 步洗手法洗手并戴口罩。

3. Prepare the equipments. Place linens on the nursing trolley in order of use.

准备用物，按使用顺序将用物置于护理车上。

4. Wash hands and remove the mask.

洗手、摘口罩。

5. Take all the equipment to the patient's bedside.

携用物至患者床旁。

6. Assess the environment. Wash hands and put on the mask.

评估环境，洗手、戴口罩。

7. Check for the bed number and patient's name. Ask the reason for going out and return time. Assist the patient to get off the bed.

核对患者床号、姓名，询问其外出原因及返回时间，协助患者下床。

8. Move the bedside chair next to the foot of the bed.

将床旁椅移至床尾。

9. Check for personal items the patient may have dropped in the bed, such as a watch.

检查患者有无手表等个人物品落在床上。

10. Check for soiled linens and replace them as needed.

检查有无已被弄脏的床上用物，根据需要进行更换。

11. Sweep the large sheet on the bed using a bed-brush with a damp cover if necessary.

必要时用带湿套的床刷清扫床大单。

12. If the corners of the bed are loosened, miter them using the same method as for "making a closed bed".

如果床角松散，则铺床角，方法同"铺备用床"。

13. Place the quilt on the bed with its vertical center fold at the vertical center line of the bed and with its top placed so that the hem is 15 cm away from the head of the bed.

将盖被放在床上，使其纵中线对齐床的纵中线，上缘距离床头 15 cm。

14. Tuck in the two side edges of the quilt along the edges of the bed and tuck in its end along the end of the bed.

将盖被两侧平齐床缘内折，尾端平齐床尾内折。

15. Infolding one quarter of the quilt and then fold the quilt down to the foot of the bed into three parts.

将盖被的四分之一向内折，再将盖被扇形三折叠于床尾。

16. Soften the pillow.

拍松枕头。

17. Place the pillow at the head of the bed with the open end of the pillowcase facing away from the door of the room.

将枕头横放于床头，枕套开口端背门。

18. Return the bedside table and chair.

移回床旁桌和床旁椅。

19. Discard all used equipment appropriately.

合理清理用物。

20. Wash hands and remove the mask.

洗手、摘口罩。

Nurse Alert 护理事项

Same as for"Making a closed bed".

同"铺备用床"。

1.3 Making a Postoperative Bed 铺麻醉床

Purpose 操作目的

1. To facilitate a postoperative patient's transfer into a bed from the operating room and receipt of treatments and nursing care.

方便术后患者转运并接受治疗和护理。

2. To provide a safe and comfortable environment for a postoperative patient in order to prevent postoperative complications.

为手术后患者提供安全、舒适的环境及预防术后并发症的发生。

3. To prevent the patient's linens from being soiled with excretions or other body discharges and facilitate their replacement.

避免床上用物被分泌物或其他体液污染，便于更换。

Assessment 评估

1. Assess the patient's diagnosis, health condition, anesthetic type, operation site and equipment for postoperative emergency as needed.

评估患者的诊断、病情、麻醉方式、手术部位及术后需要的抢救物品等。

2. Check whether other patients in the ward are receiving therapy or dining.

检查病室其他患者是否正在进行治疗或进餐。

Gather equipment 物品准备

Equipments：护理车上（由上至下）依次为 pillowcase 枕套，quilt cover 被套，rubber drawsheet 橡胶单，cloth drawsheet 中单，large sheet 大单，hand sanitizer 洗手液，bed brush 床刷，bed brush cover（if necessary）床刷套（按需准备）。

Equipment for postoperative care 术后麻醉用物：tray 治疗盘，mouth gag and tongue forceps 开口器及舌钳，tongue blade 压舌板，oropharyngeal tube 口咽通气导管，sphygmomanometer and stethoscope 血压计和听诊器，sterile bowl 无菌治疗碗，nasal catheter or cannula 鼻导管或吸氧管，sterile suction catheters 无菌吸痰管，sterile swabs 无菌棉签，sterile forceps 无菌镊子，sterile gauzes 无菌纱布，flashlight 手电筒，drape 治疗巾，kidney basin 弯盘，adhesive tape 胶布，record chart and pen 护理记录单及笔，oxygen equipment and suction equipment 吸氧与吸痰装置。

Procedure 操作过程

1. Report and tidy your dress.

报告并整理仪表。

2. Check the validity of hand sanitizer and wash hands in 7 steps and put on the mask.

检查洗手液的有效期，7 步洗手法洗手并戴口罩。

3. Assess the patient before operation（surgery site、the number of drainage tube）. Prepare the equipments according to the need and place linens on the nursing trolley in order of use.

操作前评估患者（手术部位及引流管数量）。根据术后患者的需要准备用物，按使用顺序将物品置于护理车上。

4. Wash hands and remove the mask.

洗手、摘口罩。

5. Take all the equipment to the patient's bedside.

携用物至患者床旁。

6. Assess for the environment of the ward, ensure that no patients in the ward are receiving therapy or dining.

评估病室环境，确保病室内没有患者正在进行治疗或进餐。

7. Wash hands and put on a mask.

洗手、戴口罩。

8. Move the bedside table about 20 cm away from the bed.

移开床旁桌，使其距离床约 20 cm。

9. Move the bedside chair next to the foot of the bed.

将床旁椅移至床尾。

10. Place linens on the chair in order of use.

按使用顺序将床上用物放在椅子上。

11. Strip the used sheet, quilt cover and pillowcase. Folding the pillow、mattress and quilt.

撤去用过的大单、被套及枕套。折好枕芯、床褥及棉胎。

12. Check the mattress and turn it over as needed. Move it up to the head of the bed and center it. Align the mattress pad flat out on the mattress. Sweep it using a bed-brush with a damp cover.

检查床垫并根据需要翻转床垫。将床垫往上推，居中齐床头。将床褥对齐床头平铺于床垫上，用带湿套的床刷清扫床褥。

13. Place a large sheet on the mattress with its horizontal and vertical center lines of the mattress.

将大单放在床垫上，使其横中线和纵中线对齐床垫的相应中线。

14. Unfold the large sheet in sequence from the head to the foot of the bed, from the near side to the opposite side.

从床头到床尾、从近侧到对侧依次打开大单。

15. Tuck the excess large sheet under the head of the mattress.

将床头余下部分的大单折入床垫下。

16. Make a mitered corner at the head of the bed on the near side.

铺近侧床头角。

17. Making a mitered corner: Lifts the corner of the mattress with your right

hand, and folds the rest part of the large sheet under the mattress with your left hand. Lift the edge of the large sheet 30 cm away from the head of a bed, make the lifting part looks like an equilateral triangle, and then fold two Angles under the mattress respectively.

包角：右手托起床垫一角，另一手伸过床头中线将大单折入床垫下，在距离床头约30 cm处，向上提起大单边缘，使大单头端呈等边三角形，再分别将两角塞于床垫下。

18. Move to the foot of the bed, tuck the excess large sheet under the foot of the mattress, make a mitered corner in the same way for the head of the bed on the same side.

移至床尾，将床尾余下部分的大单折入床垫下，同法包好同侧床尾角。

19. Move to the center of the bed, tuck the remainder of the large sheet's center part under the mattress.

移至床中部，将大单中部边缘塞于床垫下。

20. Lay cloth drawsheet and rubber drawsheet on the bed as needed according to the anesthetic type and operation site that the patient will receive, with their vertical center folds at the vertical center line of the bed.

根据患者的麻醉方式及手术部位将中单、橡胶单置于患者需要的位置上，使其纵中线对齐床的纵中线。

21. Unfold the cloth drawsheet and rubber drawsheet respectively, tuck the remainders of the drawsheet under the mattress.

分别将中单、橡胶单展开，将余下部分塞于床垫下。

22. Move to the opposite side of the bed, repeat steps 13-21 to make the large sheet on the opposite side. At last pull the large sheet, cloth drawsheet and rubber drawsheet toward you and straighten out the sheet to make sure that there are no wrinkles in them. Miter bed corners and tuck the sheets under the mattress.

转至床对侧，重复步骤13～21，同法铺好对侧大单。最后将大单、中单和橡胶单向一侧牵拉确保床单没有褶皱，将所有单子塞于床垫下。

23. Place the quilt cover on the bed with its vertical center fold at the vertical center line of the bed and with the top of the quilt cover placed so that the hem is 15 cm away from the head of the bed.

将被套放在床上，使其纵中线对齐床的纵中线，被套上缘距离床头15 cm。

24. Unfold the quilt cover in sequence, draw its end of upper-layer upwards from its placket.

依次打开被套，将被套尾部开口端上层向上打开1/3处。

25. Place the quilt folded in "S" form into the placket of the quilt cover so that its end is even with the end of the quilt cover.

将"S"形折叠的棉胎放入被套尾端开口处，棉胎底边与被套开口边缘平齐。

26. Pull the top of the quilt into the top of the quilt cover with your left hand.

用左手将棉胎上端拉至被套顶端。

27. Unfold the quilt and make it even with the quilt cover.

展开棉胎，使其平铺于被套内。

28. Unfold the end of the quilt and make it even with the quilt cover in the same way, tie the open end of the quilt cover.

用同样的方法展开棉胎尾部于被套内后拉平被套，系带打结。

29. Tuck in the two side edges of the quilt along the edges of the bed and tuck in its end along the end of the bed.

将盖被两侧平齐床缘内折，尾端平齐床尾内折。

30. Fan-fold the quilt to the side of the bed facing away from the door of the room.

将盖被三折叠于背门一侧，开口向门。

31. Open the pillowcase and slip it over the pillow. Tie the open end of the pillowcase.

打开枕套并套于枕芯外，系带打结。

32. Place the pillow in an upright position at the head of the bed with the open end of the pillowcase facing away from the door of the room.

将枕头横放于床头，枕套开口端背门。

33. Return the bedside table and chair so that the chair is not in the way where the postoperative patient is being transferred into the bed.

移回床旁桌和床旁椅，注意椅子的位置不要妨碍患者的术后过床。

34. Lay the equipment for postoperative care on the bedside table. Place the oxygen equipment, suction equipment and IV pole in proper places.

将术后护理用物置于床旁桌上。将吸氧与吸痰装置、输液架置于适当位置。

35. Have the call signal within patient's reach.

将呼叫器置于患者易取处。

36. Discard all used equipment appropriately.

合理清理用物。

37. Wash hands and remove the mask.

洗手、摘口罩。

Nurse Alert 护理事项

1. Lay disposable drawsheet on the bed as needed according to the anesthetic type and operation site that the patient will receive. If a rubber drawsheet is used, a cloth drawsheet should be placed over it completely, because any exposed rubber can irritate the patient's skin.

根据患者的麻醉方式及手术部位将一次性中单放于床上患者需要的位置。如果使用了橡胶单，中单必须完全盖住橡胶单，因为橡胶暴露会刺激患者的皮肤。

2. Equipment for postoperative care should meet the patient's need in order for the patient to receive first-aid and nursing care immediately.

术后护理用物应符合患者的需要，以使患者术后及时得到抢救和护理。

3. Always use good body mechanics to conserve time and energy. For example, when you place an adjustable bed in the high position and drop the bed side rails, using correct posture can reduce strain on you as you work.

运用人体力学原理以省时和节力。例如，将升降床升起、将床栏放下等动作若采取正确姿势可以减轻操作者的肌肉疲劳。

4. Smooth the bed so that it is free of wrinkles to avoid irritating patient's skin and causing discomfort.

床铺平整无褶皱，以免刺激患者皮肤及引起不适。

New Words and Expressions
单 词 表

postoperative [pəust'ɔpərətiv] *adj*. 手术后的

complication [ˌkɔmpli'keiʃən] *n*. 并发症

excretion [eks'kriːʃən] *n*. 排泄，排泄物；分泌，分泌物

discharge [dis'tʃɑːdʒ] *n*. 排出物，引流物

diagnosis [ˌdaiəg'nəusis] *n*. 诊断

anesthetic [ˌænis'θetik] *adj*. 麻醉的；感觉缺失的

emergency [i'məːdʒ (ə)nsi] *n*. 紧急情况；突发事件；非常时刻

drawsheet ['drɔːʃiːt] *n*. （住院患者用的）垫单；抽单

gag [gæg] *n*. 塞口物

forceps ['fɔːseps] *n*. [医] 钳子；医用镊子

oropharyngeal [ˈɔːrəuˌfærinˈdʒiːəl] *adj.* 口咽的
sphygmomanometer [ˌsfigməuməˈnɔmitə] *n.* 血压计
stethoscope [ˈsteθəskəup] *n.* 听诊器
nasal [ˈneizəl] *adj.* 鼻的；鼻音的
catheter [ˈkæθitə] *n.* [医] 导管；导尿管
cannula [ˈkænjulə] *n.* [医] 套管；[临床] 插管
swab [swɔb] *n.* 药签，棉签；[外科] 拭子；医用海绵，纱布；拖把
gauze [gɔːz] *n.* 纱布；薄纱
drape [dreip] *n.* 治疗巾
kidney basin 弯盘(腰形盘)
IV pole 输液架

Communication Model
沟通模板

Self-introduction Model 常规介绍模板

Good morning/afternoon teachers, my name is ××, I come from class ××, my student's number is ××. Today, I am going to show you the process of making a postoperative bed, the equipments I have prepared are ... ,everything is ready, may I start?

老师上午/下午好，我是××，来自××班，我的学号为××。今天我要展示的操作是铺麻醉床，所准备的用物有……，准备完毕，请求开始。

Assessment 评估

There is no patient receiving therapy or dining in the ward. The patient is diagnosed with appendicitis. The Surgical incision site is in the lower abdomen. The patient has been sent to the operating room. Now, I will make the postoperative bed for the patient.

病室内无人进食或接受治疗。患者已确诊为阑尾炎，手术切口位于下腹部，现已送进手术室，现在为患者铺麻醉床。

Scoring Criteria 2

评分细则 2

项目		总分	技术操作要求	标准分	扣分说明	得分
评估 10	仪表	2	仪表端庄、服装整洁、修剪指甲、洗手、戴口罩	2	一项不符扣1分	
	物品	6	用物齐备，治疗车上下放置合理	6	一项不符扣1分	
	环境	2	评估环境符合操作要求	2	一项不符扣1分	
实施 70	铺床褥	10	移开床旁桌、椅位置符合要求	2	一项不符扣1分	
			检查床垫，将其余物品放于床旁椅上	2	一项不符扣1分	
			床褥齐床头展开方法正确	2	一项不符扣1分	
			平铺床褥方法正确、平整	4	一项不符扣2分	
	铺大单 铺中单 橡胶单	28	大单放置正确，分别向床头、床尾展开	2	一项不符扣1分	
			铺近侧大单：逐层展开，折角，手法、顺序正确	4	一项不符扣1分	
			根据病情放置近侧橡胶单位置正确	4	一项不符扣2分	
			铺中单位置及展开方法正确，能覆盖橡胶单	4	一项不符扣2分	
			铺对侧大单：展开、折角，手法、顺序正确	4	一项不符扣1分	
			铺对侧橡胶单位置及展开方法正确	2	一项不符扣2分	
			铺对侧中单位置及展开方法正确，能覆盖橡胶单	2	一项不符扣2分	
			各单中线均与床中线对齐	2	一项不符扣2分	
			床角及边缘整齐、紧扎、美观	2	一项不符扣1分	
			床面平整、美观	2	一项不符扣1分	
	套被套	20	被套位置正确、一次展开	2	一项不符扣1分	
			棉胎放置合理、展开方法正确	4	一项不符扣2分	
			被套两侧对称、齐床沿	2	一项不符扣1分	
			被套中线与床中线齐	2	一项不符扣2分	
			被尾折叠平整、齐床尾，系带无外露	4	一项不符扣2分	
			被头充实，距床头适宜(15 cm)	2	一项不符扣1分	
			被套三折于背门一侧	4	一项不符扣2分	
	套枕套	6	在床尾或椅子上套枕套，方法正确	2	一项不符扣2分	
			枕头四角平整、充实	1	一项不符扣1分	
			系带打结	1	一项不符扣1分	
			枕头摆放方式正确，开口背门	2	一项不符扣2分	
	整理	6	移回床旁桌，动作轻稳	2	一项不符扣1分	
			床旁椅放背门一侧	2	一项不符扣2分	
			用物处理正确，洗手	2	一项不符扣2分	
评价 20	能力	6	铺床中部橡胶单、中单上缘距离床头45～50 cm	4	一项不符扣2分	
			按规定时间完成(6 min)	2	每超过30 s扣1分	
	英语	10	发音准确，语言流畅，关爱患者，符合逻辑	10	一项不符扣2分	
	效果	4	床单位整体符合要求，护士操作符合力学原理	4	一项不符扣2分	
主考教师签字：			日期：	总分：100	得分：	

评分标准：91～100分为优，81～90分为良，71～80分为中，60～70分为差，低于60分为不及格。

1.4 Changing an Occupied Bed
卧床患者更换床单法

Purpose 操作目的

1. To keep the hospital bed neat and make the patients comfortable.

保持患者床单位整洁，使患者感觉舒适。

2. To prevent complications such as pressure ulcer.

预防压疮等并发症发生。

Assessment 评估

1. Assess the patient's age, gender, body weight and health condition, such as level of consciousness, impaired physical mobility, hemiplegia, paraplegia, fracture, presence of drainage tubes, infusion tubes, wound, bowel or urinary incontinence.

评估患者的年龄、性别、体重及病情，如意识状态、有无躯体移动障碍、偏瘫、截瘫和骨折，有无引流管、输液管及伤口，有无大小便失禁等。

2. Assess the cleanliness of the patient's linens.

评估患者床上用物的清洁程度。

3. Assess the patient's psychological status, ability to cooperate and communication skills.

评估患者的心理状态、合作程度及表达能力。

4. Check whether other patients in the ward are receiving therapy or dining.

检查病室内其他患者是否正在进行治疗或进餐。

Gather equipment 物品准备

Equipments:护理车上(由上至下)依次为 large sheet 大单，cloth drawsheet 中单，quilt cover 被套，pillowcase 枕套，bed-brush 床刷，clean clothing (if necessary)清洁衣裤(按需准备)，linen hamper for soiled linens 污衣袋，hand sanitizer 洗手液。

Procedure 操作过程

1. Report and tidy your dress.

报告并整理仪表。

2. Check the validity of hand sanitizer and wash hands in 7 steps and put on the mask.

检查洗手液的有效期,7 步洗手法洗手并戴口罩。

3. Prepare the equipments. Place linens on the nursing trolley in order of use.

准备用物,按使用顺序将用物置于护理车上。

4. Wash hands and remove the mask.

洗手、摘口罩。

5. Take the equipments to the patient's bedside. Assess the environment. Check for the bed number and patient's name. Explain the purpose of the procedure to obtain patient's consent.

携用物至患者床旁。评估环境,核对患者床号、姓名并解释操作目的以取得患者同意。

6. Tell the patient to inform nurse of any discomfort during the procedure.

告知患者在操作过程中若有不适立即汇报。

7. Close the door and windows.

关闭门窗。

8. Open the cap of garbage bin. Wash hands and put on the mask.

打开污物桶盖,洗手、戴口罩。

9. Move the bedside table about 20 cm away from the bed.

移开床旁桌使其距离床约 20 cm。

10. Move the bedside chair next to the foot of the bed.

将床旁椅移至床尾。

11. Move the nursing trolley about 15 cm away from the end of the bed.

将护理车置于距离床尾约 15 cm 的位置。

12. Make the bed flat if permitted, push the mattress to the head of the bed.

如果病情许可,将床放平,使床垫平床头。

13. Lower the side rail if needed and raise the side rail immediately after procedure to ensure patient's safety as he/she rolls to the edge of the bed.

根据需要放下床栏,操作后及时竖起床栏,以确保患者翻身时安全。

14. Loosen the drainage tubes fastened to the bed and place them well to avoid being pulled out.

松开固定在床上的各种引流管并妥善处理，以防脱落。

15. Loosen the quilt. Move the pillow to the opposite side of the bed.

松盖被，移枕至对侧。

16. Assist the patient to the opposite side of the bed, place him/her in side-lying position facing away from you. Advise the conscious patient to hold on the edge of the bed to protect himself/herself from falling. Assist the patient to comfortable position.

协助患者移向对侧，使其背向操作者侧卧。指导清醒患者抓住床缘防止发生坠床。协助患者取舒适体位。

17. Loosen the bottom linens on your side from the head to the foot of the bed.

从床头至床尾松开近侧各层底单。

18. Roll the soiled cloth drawsheet and large sheet upward to the center line of the bed under the patient.

上卷污中单、污大单至床中线处，塞于患者身下。

19. Sweep the mattress pad of the near side.

清扫近侧床褥。

20. Place a clean large sheet on the mattress pad and unfold the near side with its horizontal and vertical center folds in the center lines of the mattress. Roll the clean large sheet of the opposite side downward to the center line of the bed under the patient.

将清洁大单放在近侧床褥上，逐层展开，使其横中线和纵中线对齐床垫的横中线和纵中线。将对侧清洁大单内卷至床中线处，塞于患者身下。

21. Make the bed surface tight, and then make the mitered corner.

拉紧床面，包角。

22. Place a clean disposable cloth drawsheet on the mattress and unfold the near side with its vertical center fold in the center line of the mattress. Roll the clean disposable cloth drawsheet of the opposite side downward to the center line of the bed under the patient.

将清洁的一次性中单放在床垫上并展开近侧，使其纵中线对齐床垫的纵中线，将其对侧内卷至床中线处，塞于患者身下。

23. Tuck the remaining disposable cloth drawsheet well under the mattress.

将一次性中单边缘塞入床垫下。

24. Help the patient to supine position and move the pillow to the near side of the

bed.

协助患者平卧，将枕头移至近侧。

25. Assist the patient to the near side of the bed, place him/her in side-lying position facing you. Advise the conscious patient to hold on the edge of the bed. Assist the patient to comfortable position

协助患者移至近侧，患者面向操作者侧卧。指导清醒患者手扶床边。协助患者取舒适体位。

26. Move to the opposite side of the bed.

操作者转至床对侧。

27. Loosen the bottom linens on the opposite side of the bed.

松开对侧的各层底单。

28. Roll the soiled cloth drawsheet and large sheet into a bundle respectively and discard them.

分别将污中单及污大单内卷成团并撤去。

29. Sweep the mattress pad of the opposite side.

清扫对侧床褥。

30. Making the offside large sheet: spread the clean large sheet on the mattress pad and then make the mitered corner.

铺对侧大单：展开清洁大单，拉平并包好床角。

31. Spread the clean cloth drawsheet and tuck the remaining well under the mattress of the opposite side.

展开清洁中单并将其边缘塞入对侧床垫下。

32. Help the patient to supine position and adjust the pillow to the center of the bed.

协助患者取仰卧位，将枕头移至床中间。

33. Place the clean quilt cover over the soiled one, fold the quilt into "S" form in the quilt cover, and then take it out.

将清洁被套铺于污被套上逐层展开，将棉胎在被套内呈"S"形折叠取出。

34. Place the quilt into the clean quilt cover, spread the quilt and tie the cover.

将棉胎装入清洁被套内，展开铺平被套并系带打结。

35. Pull the soiled quilt cover and discard it in the lower section of the cart or into the linen hamper.

撤去污被套，放在治疗车下层或放入污衣袋内。

36. Tuck in the two side edges of the quilt along the edges of the bed and tuck in

its end along the end of the bed (or according to local policy).

将盖被两侧平齐床缘内折,尾端平齐床尾内折(或按当地要求)。

37. Remove the pillow from the bed, and change the pillowcase.

取出患者所用的枕头,更换枕套。

38. Soften the pillow and place it under the patient's bed with the open end of the pillowcase facing away from the door of the room.

将枕头拍松垫于患者头下,使其开口背门。

39. Observe the patient's health condition and the drainage tubes during the procedure. Be aware of the patient's safety, keep the patient warm and provide privacy.

全程观察患者病情及引流管情况,注意安全、保暖及保护患者的隐私。

40. Tell the patient to inform nurse immediately whenever the linens and clothing are soiled with excretions or other body discharges.

告知患者被服一旦被排泄物或引流物污染,应及时通知护士更换。

41. Instruct the patient how to use call signal and have it within patient's reach.

指导患者呼叫器的用法,并置于易取处。

42. Assist the patient to comfortable position and tidy up or change patient's clothing if necessary.

协助患者取舒适体位,必要时整理或更换衣服。

43. Fasten the drainage tubes.

固定各种引流管。

44. Replace the bedside table and chair.

移回床旁桌和床旁椅。

45. Open the door and windows.

打开门窗。

46. Discard all used equipment appropriately.

整理用物。

47. Close the garbage cap. Wash hands and remove the mask.

关污物桶盖,洗手、摘口罩。

Nurse Alert 护理事项

1. While making the bed, there should be no other patients in the ward receiving therapy or dining.

铺床时,病室内没有其他患者正在进行治疗或进餐。

2. Always use good body mechanics to conserve time and energy.

运用人体力学原理以省时和节力。

3. Be aware of the patient's safety, keep the patient warm, provide privacy and observe the patient's health condition.

能注意安全、保暖及保护患者的隐私，注意观察患者的病情。

4. If a rubber drawsheet is used, a cloth drawsheet should be placed over it completely, because any exposed rubber can irritate the patient's skin.

如果使用了橡胶单，中单必须完全覆盖橡胶单，因为橡胶暴露会刺激患者皮肤。

5. The bed is made smooth, clean and free of wrinkles to avoid irritating the patient's skin and causing discomfort.

床铺应平整、清洁、无褶皱，以免刺激患者皮肤及引起不适。

6. For a patient who is critically ill, with many tubes, with spinal trauma or receiving spinal operation, it is necessary to change an occupied bed by more than two nurses.

病情重、全身管道多、脊柱损伤或脊柱手术的患者应两人以上协同更换床单。

7. Avoid shaking the linens to prevent the spread of microorganisms and dust particles. Sweep the mattress using a bed-brush with a damp cover. One bed-brush cover can only be used for one mattress.

避免抖动床单，以防病原微生物播散并防止尘埃飞扬。使用带湿套的床刷清扫床垫。一个床刷套只扫一张床垫。

8. Dispose of soiled linens and clothing in the lower section of the cart or into the linen hamper. Do not place them on the floor or on another patient's bed.

污被服应放在治疗车下层或放入污衣袋中，不可放在地板上或其他患者的病床上。

New Words and Expressions
单 词 表

complication [ˌkɔmpliˈkeiʃən] *n.* 并发症

consciousness [ˈkɔnʃəsnis] *n.* 意识；知觉；觉悟；感觉

hemiplegia [ˌhemiˈpliːdʒiə] *n.* [内科] 偏瘫，半身麻痹；[中医] 半身不遂

paraplegia [ˌpærəˈpliːdʒiə] *n.* [内科] 截瘫，半身不遂

fracture [ˈfræktʃə] *n.* 骨折

drainage [ˈdreinidʒ] *n.* 引流物、排出液

Communication Model
沟 通 模 板

Self-introduction Model 常规介绍模板

Good morning/afternoon teachers, my name is ××, I come from class ××, my student's number is ××. Today, I am going to show you the process of changing an occupied bed, the equipments I have prepared are. . . ,everything is ready, may I start?

老师上午/下午好,我是××,来自××班,我的学号为××。今天我要展示的操作是卧床患者更换床单,所准备的用物有……,准备完毕,请求开始。

Assessment 评估

The ward is tidy and well ventilated. There is no patient are receiving therapy or dining in the ward. The patient has surgical incision in the abdomen and he can not rotate by himself. The patient is in good mental state, he can cooperate with me.

病室整洁,通风良好。无患者正在进行治疗或进餐。患者腹部有手术切口不能自行翻身。患者精神状态良好,能予以配合。

Communication 沟通

Good morning, sir. May I have your full name please? OK. Mr ××, I'm your duty nurse today, you can call me ××. How do you feel now? You haven't changed your linens more than one week after the operation, and I am going to change it for you. Don't worry, I know you can't get up right now, and I can do it in special way. Would you please cooperate with me when I need your help? Thank you, do you need to use a bedpan to empty your bladder now? OK, I have to turn you lying on the left or right side in the procedure. So, if you have any discomfort, please let me know and I'll do it gently.

早上好,先生。请问您的名字是什么? 您好,××先生。我是您今天的责任护士,您可以叫我××,您感觉怎么样了? 您已经一周多没有更换床单了,我将为您更换。我知道您现在还不能起床,不用担心,我会用特别的方法。您可以在我需要您帮助的时候配合我吗？谢谢，您现在需要方便一下吗？好的，在操作中我可能需要您向左或向右翻身，如果在过程中您有任何不适，请告诉我，我会动作很轻柔的。

Now I'll turn you to left-side lying position. Please raise your head and flex your right knee. Pay attention to softening your belly without forcing. OK, very good. Hold on the edge of the bed with your hands.

现在我要帮您取左侧卧位，请您抬头并曲右膝。注意保持腹部放松。很好，请您双手握住床栏。

It is time to turn right.

现在取右侧卧位。

Let's change the quilt cover. Would you please help me holding the two corners with your hands? Thank you.

现在来更换被套。请您帮我抓住被套的两角，谢谢。

I'll change pillowcase, so I have to remove the pillow from your head. OK, raise your head again.

接下来要换枕套，所以需要将枕头移开，好的，请抬头。

Your linens is clear, if you need any help, please inform me immediately. You can press the button on the call signal. I'll come here as soon as possible. Have a good rest!

您的床单位现在很干净，如果您需要帮助，请立即通知我。您可以按呼叫器，我会尽快赶来。好好休息！

Scoring Criteria 3
评分细则 3

项目		总分	技术操作要求	标准分	扣分说明	得分
评估 10	仪表	2	仪表端庄、服装整洁、修剪指甲、洗手、戴口罩	2	一项不符扣1分	
	物品	4	用物备齐，放置合理	2	一项不符扣1分	
	环境		环境清洁、安静(酌情关闭门窗或屏风遮挡)	2	一项不符扣1分	
	评估	4	了解患者病情、意识状态、心理状态及自理能力	4	一项不符扣1分	
实施 70	核对	4	核对床号、姓名	2	一项不符扣1分	
	解释		解释操作目的、过程及配合方法	2	一项不符扣1分	
	更换大单中单	30	移开床旁桌和床旁椅位置得当、动作轻稳	2	一项不符扣1分	
			松被尾、床单方法正确	2	一项不符扣1分	
			移枕头，协助患者翻身动作轻稳	4	一项不符扣2分	
			清扫床褥方法正确(干式)	2	一项不符扣2分	
			换从大单到中单顺序、手法正确	8	一项不符扣2分	
			大单、中单平整，四角扎紧，中线正	6	一项不符扣1分	
			污单取出得当(污染面不接触清洁单的清洁面)	4	一项不符扣1分	
			放置合理(污染被服不落地)	2	一项不符扣2分	
	更换被套	24	更换步骤、方法正确	6	一项不符扣1分	
			被套、棉胎内外平整、美观	4	一项不符扣1分	
			被头端无虚边、被尾折叠平整齐床尾，系带无外露	6	一项不符扣2分	
			被套对称、两侧齐床沿，中线正	4	一项不符扣1分	
			取污被套方法正确、放置合理	4	一项不符扣2分	
	更换枕套	6	更换方法正确	2	一项不符扣2分	
			四角充实、外观平整	2	一项不符扣1分	
			枕头放置位置正确、开口背门	2	一项不符扣1分	
	整理	6	移回床旁桌和床旁椅，动作轻稳	2	一项不符扣1分	
			床单位整洁，开窗通风	2	一项不符扣1分	
			用物处理正确，洗手	2	一项不符扣1分	
评价 20	熟练	6	操作轻稳、熟练，步骤合理	2	一项不符扣1分	
			相关理论知识掌握熟练	2	酌情扣分	
			按规定时间完成(15 min)	2	酌情扣分	
	效果	4	患者感觉安全、保暖、舒适，无导管、辅料等脱落	4	酌情扣分	
	英语	10	关爱患者，沟通有效；英语发音标准，语言流畅，符合操作场景要求	10	酌情扣分	
主考教师：			日期：	总分：100	得分：	

评分标准：91～100分为优，81～90分为良，71～80分为中，60～70分为差，低于60分为不及格。

注：换单时若发生患者坠床、导管或辅料脱落等，该项考核为不及格。

Chapter 2
Special Mouth Care
特殊口腔护理

Purpose　操作目的

1. To keep the patient's mouth clean and moist in order to prevent oral complications such as oral infection.

保持口腔清洁和湿润，预防口腔感染等并发症。

2. To prevent or minimize halitosis or to remove plaque on the surfaces of the teeth in order to keep the patient comfortable.

预防或减轻口腔异味，清除牙垢，保持患者舒适。

3. To monitor changes in the patient's health condition by observing oral condition.

通过观察口腔情况监测患者的病情变化。

Assessment　评估

1. Assess the patient's age, level of consciousness, and health condition including whether he/she has received operation, has a retention of nasogastric tube, endotracheal intubation or tracheal cannula, and whether he/she is receiving chemotherapy or radiotherapy.

评估患者的年龄、意识及病情，包括有无手术，有无留置胃管、气管插管或气管套管，是否正在进行化疗或放疗。

2. Assess for clearness and any abnormalities in the patient's mouth.

评估患者口腔的卫生状况及各种异常情况。

(1) Assess the patient's lips, noting whether they are dry, cracked or bleeding.

评估患者的口唇情况,注意有无干裂或出血。

(2) Assess the condition of the patient's teeth, noting any decay and whether he/she wears dentures.

评估患者的牙齿情况,注意有无龋齿及义齿。

(3) Assess the condition of the patient's gums, mucous membranes and tongue, noting whether there are any ulcers, any inflammation, swelling or bleeding, the presence of any halitosis.

评估患者的牙龈、口腔黏膜及舌的情况,注意口腔有无水疱、溃疡,有无炎症、肿胀或出血,有无口臭。

(4) Assess the palate and the underside of the patient's tongue.

评估患者的上腭及舌底。

3. Assess the patient's psychological status, ability to cooperate, communication skills, self-care ability and knowledge of oral hygiene.

评估患者的心理状态、合作态度、表达能力、自理能力及口腔卫生知识水平。

Gather equipment 物品准备

治疗盘(medication tray)内:bowl 治疗碗 2 个(分别盛 mouth wash 漱口液和sterile balls 无菌棉球),forceps 镊子,curved hemostat forceps 弯止血钳,kidney basin 弯盘,tongue blade 压舌板,drinking straw 吸水管,swabs 棉签,liquid paraffin 液体石蜡,flashlight 手电筒,gauzes 纱布数块,towel/cloth(if necessary)治疗巾(按需准备),mouth gag 开口器。

治疗盘外:mouth wash 常用漱口液,medication (if necessary)口腔外用药(按需准备),hand sanitizer 洗手液。治疗车下层备:garbage bin 生活垃圾桶,medical garbage bin 医用垃圾桶。

Procedure 操作过程

1. Report and tidy your dress.

报告并整理仪表。

2. Check the validity of hand sanitizer and wash hands in 7 steps and put on the mask.

检查洗手液的有效期，7步洗手法洗手并戴口罩。

3. Prepare the equipments.

准备用物。

4. Wash hands and remove the mask.

洗手、摘口罩。

5. Take the equipment to the bedside. Evaluate the environment of the ward.

携用物到患者床旁。评估病室环境是否适宜操作。

6. Check the patient's bed number and name. Explain the purpose for the operation.

核对患者床号和姓名。解释操作目的。

7. Assist the patient to lateral position or lying on back with the patient's head turned to one side and facing you.

协助患者取侧卧位或仰卧位，使其头偏向一侧，面向操作者。

8. Place a cloth under the patient's chin to protect his/her gown and pillow.

颌下铺治疗巾以保护患者衣服及枕头。

9. Place a basin near the corner of the patient's mouth.

放弯盘于患者口角旁。

10. Assist the conscious patient to rinse the mouth with mouth wash using a straw and explain that this should not be swallowed. Do not let an unconscious patient rinse the mouth.

协助清醒患者用吸管吸漱口液漱口，告诉患者不要吞下漱口液。昏迷患者禁忌漱口。

11. If the patient's lips are dry and cracked, moisten them first.

如果患者口唇干裂，应先湿润口唇。

12. Assess the condition of the patient's mouth using a flashlight and a tongue blade. For an unconscious patient, open his/her mouth with a mouth gag.

使用手电筒和压舌板观察患者的口腔情况。昏迷患者可用开口器协助张口。

13. If the patient has dentures, remove and place them in a labeled cup with tap water.

如果患者有义齿，取下义齿并放于贴有标签的冷水杯中。

14. Hold a cotton ball soaked with mouth wash and remove excess mouth wash using hemostat forceps, brush the mouth orderly using one cotton ball at a time.

用止血钳夹取浸透漱口液的棉球并拧干，按顺序擦洗口腔，每次夹取一个。

(1) Ask the patient to close his/her upper and lower teeth, lift the left cheek of

the mouth with a tongue blade gently, brush the external surfaces of the left teeth lengthways from the molar to the central incisor. Brush the right side in the same way.

患者咬合上、下牙齿,用压舌板轻轻撑开左侧颊部,沿纵向擦洗左侧的外表面,由臼齿向门齿。同法擦洗右侧。

(2) Ask the patient to separate his/her upper and lower teeth, brush the inner surfaces and crowns' tips of the left upper teeth, then the inner surfaces and crowns' tips of the left lower teeth lengthways; brush the left cheek with a rotating action. Brush the right side in the same way.

嘱患者张开牙齿,沿纵向擦洗牙齿的左上内侧面、左上咬合面、左下内侧面、左下咬合面,弧形擦洗左侧颊部。同法擦洗右侧。

(3) Brush the hard palate, the surface and underside of the tongue breadthwise.

横向擦洗硬腭、舌面及舌底。

15. Assist the conscious patient to rinse the mouth again with a drinking straw and then spit the fluid into the basin, dry the lips with a piece of tissue.

协助清醒患者用吸管吸水再次漱口,然后将漱口水吐到弯盘中,用纸巾擦净口唇。

16. Inspect the mouth for clearness or any trauma.

检查口腔的清洁效果及有无损伤。

17. If the lips are dry, apply a thin layer of liquid paraffin or lip balm to the patient's lips. If there is ulcer or bleeding, apply external medication as ordered.

如果口唇干燥,可涂上一薄层液体石蜡或润唇膏。若有口腔溃疡或出血,则遵医嘱用药。

18. Tell the patient the importance of good oral hygiene, and introduce oral hygiene knowledge to prevent oral complications.

告知患者保持口腔卫生的重要性,向其介绍口腔护理的相关知识,以预防各种口腔并发症。

19. Ask the patient to notify nurse immediately whenever any unusual effects are occurring.

告知患者若有不适立即告知护士。

20. Instruct the patient how to use call signal and have it within patient's reach.

指导患者呼叫器的用法,并置于易取处。

21. Assist the patient to comfortable position and tidy up clothing if necessary.

协助患者取舒适体位,必要时整理衣服。

22. Ask the patient's feelings and needs.

询问患者的感受及需求。

23. Tidy up the patient's bed.

整理床单位。

24. Discard all used equipment appropriately.

合理清理用物。

25. Remove gloves, if used. Wash hands and remove the mask.

脱手套(如有使用),洗手、摘口罩。

26. Sign the treatment sheet or nursing care plan to indicate that the special mouth care has been administered.

在治疗单或护理计划单上签名,表示特殊口腔护理已执行。

27. Document any abnormalities about the patient's oral condition and the effectiveness of mouth care in the nursing record.

在护理记录单上记录患者的口腔异常情况及口腔护理的效果。

Nurse Alert 护理事项

1. For an unconscious patient, no month rinsing is allowed in order to avoid aspiration.

昏迷患者禁忌漱口,以免引起误吸。

2. Open the mouth of an unconscious patient with a mouth gag. Firstly, separate his/her upper and lower teeth carefully with a metal tongue blade wrapped with gauze, then insert the mouth gag wrapped with gauze gently between the back molars. Do not force.

用开口器协助昏迷患者张口。先用缠绕纱布的金属压舌板分开患者上、下牙齿,然后轻轻将开口器从臼齿处放入。切忌用力过猛。

3. Brush the patient's mouth with cotton balls soaked with mouthwash, each cotton ball should be dried using hemostat forceps moderately to avoid aspiration.

用含漱口液的棉球擦洗口腔,每个棉球应使用止血钳拧干,防止误吸。

4. Hold each cotton ball using hemostat forceps, brush one placeat a time to avoid leaving cotton balls in the mouth. The tip of the hemostat forceps should be wrapped with a cotton ball thoroughly and be used gently to avoid injuring the mucous membranes and gums.

止血钳每次夹一个棉球,一个棉球擦洗一个部位,以防棉球遗留在口腔内。棉球应包裹止血钳尖端。擦洗时动作宜轻柔,防止碰伤黏膜及牙龈。

5. For patients who receive frequent antibiotics therapy, observe epiphyte

infection in the mouth.

对长期使用抗生素的患者，观察其口腔内是否有真菌感染。

New Words and Expressions
单 词 表

consciousness [ˈkɔnʃəsnis] *n.* 意识；知觉；感觉
nasogastric tube 鼻胃管；胃管
endotracheal intubation 气管插管
tracheal cannula 气管套管
denture [ˈdentʃə] *n.* 假牙；补齿(常用复数)
mucous membrane 黏膜
sterile [ˈsterail] *adj.* 无菌的
forceps [ˈfɔːseps] *n.* [医]钳子；医用镊子
liquid paraffin 液体石蜡
rotating action 原意为旋转动作，在此引申为弧形擦洗

Communication
沟 通

Self-introduction Model 常规介绍模板

Good morning/afternoon teachers, my name is ××, I come from class ××, my student's number is ××. Today, I am going to show you the process of special mouth care, the equipments I have prepared are ... ,everything is ready, may I start?

老师上午/下午好，我是××，来自××班，我的学号为××。今天我要展示的操作是口腔护理，所准备的用物有……，准备完毕，请求开始。

Assessment 评估

The ward is tidy and well ventilated. The patient is in good mental state, he can open his mouth. There is no abnormalities in the patient's mouth but a lot of secretion.

病室整洁、通风良好。患者精神状态良好，能够自己张嘴，口腔内有较多分泌物但无其他异常情况。

Communication　沟通

Hello, I'm your duty nurse, my name is ××. Would you tell me your full name, please? Because of the nasogastric feeding, you do not need to eat through the mouth, it is really a risk factor for oral infection. In order to prevent infection, I am going to give you a special mouth care and you will feel comfortable after that.

您好，我是您今天的责任护士，我叫××，能告诉我您的名字吗？由于您使用鼻胃管进食，不能正常经口腔咀嚼食物，这是一个容易诱发口腔感染的因素。现在我要为您做口腔护理来避免出现感染，做完后您会觉得很舒适的。

I'll turn you to the lateral position(right-side lying position) or supine position with your head facing me.

请转身侧卧或平卧，头朝向我这一边。

Please rinse your mouth and spit the water into the kidney basin.

请吸水漱口，将水吐到弯盘内。

Please open your mouth(open up). Let me check the condition of your mouth. Do you have any dentures or ulcer in your mouth? (take up the flashlight)①Yes—please take it out and I'll keep it for you. ②No—OK, there are no dentures, ulcers, swelling or bleeding. OK, very well.

好的，请张开嘴让我来帮您检查一下口腔的状况。您有活动的义齿或口腔溃疡吗？(点亮手电筒，用手遮挡患者眼睛)①有——请拿下来我暂时帮您保存。②没有——好的，您口腔中没有义齿、溃疡、肿胀或出血，非常适合操作。

Would you please close your upper and lower teeth?

请咬合您的上、下牙齿。

OK, open your teeth now. I will scrub the teeth for you.

好，现在请张开嘴，我要为您擦拭牙齿。

I'll brush the underside of the tongue, now please up your tongue.

现在我要刷洗您的舌下部位，请将舌头抬起来。

Please rinse your mouth again and spit the water into the kidney basin.

请再次吸水漱口，将水吐到弯盘内。

Open the mouth and I'll check your month again. OK, well done.

张开嘴巴，让我再检查一下口腔，非常好。

I'll give you lip balm to keep your lips moist.

我来帮您涂上润唇膏吧,它能帮您保持嘴唇的湿润状态。

Your teeth are clean. You feel comfortable, right? I'm very happy to hear that. OK, do you feel comfortable in this position? OK, if you need any help, please press the button on the call signal. I'll come here as soon as possible. Have a good rest. See you.

现在您的口腔清洁了,感觉舒适多了吧? 很高兴听您这么说。您这个体位舒适吗? 好的,如果您有任何不适请按呼叫器找我,我会尽快过来帮助您的,好好休息,一会见。

Scoring Criteria 4
评分细则 4

项目		总分	技术操作要求	标准分	扣分说明	得分
评估13	仪表	4	仪表端庄、服装整洁、修剪指甲、洗手、戴口罩	4	一项不符扣2分	
	物品	5	根据病情准备用物，用物齐备，放置合理	3	一项不符扣1分	
	环境		环境符合操作要求	2	一项不符扣2分	
	患者	4	了解患者病情、意识状态、合作程度、口腔状况	4	一项不符扣1分	
实施63	核对解释	5	核对床号、姓名	2	一项不符扣1分	
			根据病情解释口腔护理的目的、过程、配合方法	3	一项不符扣1分	
	漱口及评估	20	根据病情摆体位(口述昏迷患者摆体位方法)	2	一项不符扣1分	
			颌下铺巾、置弯盘位置适当	4	一项不符扣2分	
			核对用物有效期、打开治疗盘正确	4	一项不符扣2分	
			及时处理口唇干裂	2	一项不符扣2分	
			漱口方式正确	2	一项不符扣2分	
			评估口腔情况(口述评估内容)	4	一项不符扣2分	
			正确使用压舌板、用后放置位置正确	2	一项不符扣1分	
	擦洗口腔	28	擦洗顺序正确，一处一个棉球	14	一项不符扣1分	
			更换棉球时无菌操作并拧干棉球	4	一项不符扣2分	
			擦洗方法正确(牙齿的外侧、内侧、咀嚼面、颊部)	4	一项不符扣1分	
			再次漱口方法正确	2	一项不符扣2分	
			再次观察口腔情况	2	一项不符扣2分	
			用纱布擦净面部	2	一项不符扣2分	
	整理	10	协助患者取舒适体位	2	一项不符扣1分	
			床单位整洁	2	一项不符扣2分	
			用物处理正确，洗手，记录	6	一项不符扣2分	
评价24	熟练	10	操作轻稳、熟练	4	一项不符扣2分	
			相关理论知识掌握熟练	2	酌情扣分	
			按规定时间完成(5min)	4	每超过30 s扣1分	
	效果	4	患者口腔清洁，感觉安全舒适，无不良反应	4	酌情扣分	
	沟通	10	关爱患者，沟通有效；英语发音标准，语言流畅，符合操作场景要求	10	酌情扣分	
主考教师签字：			日期：	总分:100	得分：	

评分标准：91～100分为优，81～90分为良，71～80分为中，60～70分为差，低于60分为不及格。

Chapter 3
Aseptic Technique
无 菌 技 术

3.1 Handling Sterile Transfer Forceps
无菌持物钳/镊的使用

Purpose 操作目的

Sterile transfer forceps are used to fetch or move a sterile item from one place to another.

无菌持物钳/镊用于取放和传递无菌物品。

Assessment 评估

1. Assess the working environment to determine whether it is in accordance with the principles of aseptic techniques.

评估操作环境是否符合无菌技术操作原则。

2. Assess the type of sterile items and their locations in order to select an appropriate sterile transfer forceps.

评估需夹取的无菌物品的种类及其放置的位置,以选择合适的无菌持物钳/镊。

3. Assess the storage method for the sterile transfer forceps (single-packaged, kept in a dry sterile container or in solution).

评估无菌持物钳/镊的保存方法(独立包装、干式或湿式保存)。

Gather equipment 物品准备

hand sanitizer 洗手液。

sterile transfer forceps 无菌持物钳/镊。可分为如下三类:① three-forked forceps 三叉钳;② oval forceps 卵圆钳;③ long or short sterile forceps 长、短镊子。sterile container 无菌容器。

Procedure 操作过程

1. Report and tidy your dress.

报告并整理仪表。

2. Check the validity of hand sanitizer and wash hands in 7 steps and put on the mask.

检查洗手液的有效期,7 步洗手法洗手并戴口罩。

3. Prepare the equipments. Place equipments on the table in order of use.

准备用物,按使用顺序将用物置于处置桌上。

4. Check the sterilization effect and expiration date of a prepared sterile transfer forceps in its container.

检查存放在容器内的无菌持物钳/镊的灭菌效果及有效期。

5. Open the cover of the container where the sterile transfer forceps are kept.

将存放无菌持物钳/镊的容器盖打开。

6. Hold the upper 1/3 part of the sterile transfer forceps, keep the tips of the forceps together and move it to the center of the container, then take it out vertically.

手持无菌持物钳/镊的上 1/3 处,闭合其前端,将其移至容器中央,然后垂直取出。

7. Close the cover of the container.

关闭容器盖。

8. Keep the tips of wet forceps downward at all times, do not reverse the direction in order to avoid the disinfectant solution flowing backward and contaminating the forceps tips.

湿无菌持物钳/镊应保持其前端向下,不可倒转,以防消毒液反流污染其前端。

9. Hold sterile transfer forceps and keep hands in front of you and from the waist to eye level. Do not reach across the sterile field.

持无菌持物钳/镊时,手应保持在身体前面、腰部以上及视线范围内。勿跨越无菌区。

10. After use, keep the tips of the forceps together, open the cover of the container, and put the forceps back into the container immediately and vertically from the center of the container, close the cover of the container.

使用后,闭合无菌持物钳/镊前端,打开容器盖,立即从容器中央垂直放回容器中,关闭容器盖。

11. Loosen the joint pivot of the sterile transfer forceps when soaking the forceps in solution.

如果是湿式保存法,应将无菌持物钳/镊的轴节松开。

New Words and Expressions
单 词 表

fetch [fetʃ] *vt.* 取来
aseptic [eiˈseptik] *adj.* 无菌的;防腐性的
sanitizer [ˈsænitaizə] *n.* 消毒杀菌剂,洗手液
oval [ˈəuvəl] *n.* 椭圆形;卵形 *adj.* 椭圆的;卵形的
sterilization [ˌsterilaiˈzeiʃən] *n.* 消毒
expiration [ˌekspəˈreiʃən] *n.* 终结
vertically [ˈvəːtikli] *adv.* 垂直地
reverse [riˈvəːs] *vt.* 颠倒;倒转
disinfectant [ˌdisinˈfektənt] *n.* 消毒剂 *adj.* 消毒的
contaminate [kənˈtæmiˌneit] *vt.* 污染
loosen [ˈluːsn] *vt.* 放松;松开
joint [dʒɔint] *n.* 关节;接合处
pivot [ˈpivət] *n.* 枢轴;中心点
soak [səuk] *vi.* 浸泡

Nurse Alert 护理事项

1. Do not use sterile transfer forceps for oily gauze in case the oil adheres to the forceps tips and affects the disinfection effect. Do not use sterile transfer forceps to do dressing or disinfect skin to prevent contamination.

不可使用无菌持物钳/镊夹取油纱布,防止油黏附于其前端而影响灭菌效果;不可

使用无菌持物钳/镊换药或消毒皮肤，以防被污染。

2. If fetching the sterile items that are far away in distance, bring the forceps together with the container to the item and use the forceps nearby.

到远处夹取无菌物品时，应将无菌持物钳/镊与其存放容器一起移至操作处，就地使用。

3. Once suspected or confirmed contamination occurs, change the sterile transfer forceps immediately.

无菌持物钳/镊一经污染或可疑污染应立即更换。

3.2 Applying Sterile Containers 无菌容器的使用

Purpose 操作目的

Sterile containers are used to conserve sterile items and keep them aseptic.

无菌容器用于盛放无菌物品以保持其无菌状态。

Assessment 评估

1. Assess the working environment to determine whether it is in accordance with the principles of aseptic techniques.

评估操作环境是否符合无菌技术操作原则。

2. Check the type, sterilization and expiration date, sterilization effect of the sterile container.

检查无菌容器的类型、灭菌日期、有效期及灭菌效果。

Gather equipment 物品准备

Equipments: hand sanitizer 洗手液，sterile container 无菌容器，sterile transfer forceps 无菌持物钳/镊，sterile bowls 无菌治疗碗，cotton balls 棉球，gauzes 纱布。

Procedure 操作过程

1. Report and tidy your dress.

报告并整理仪表。

2. Check the validity of hand sanitizer and wash hands in 7 steps and put on the mask.

检查洗手液的有效期，7 步洗手法洗手并戴口罩。

3. Prepare the equipments. Place equipments on the table in order of use.

准备用物，按使用顺序将用物置于处置桌上。

4. Check the name, sterilization and expiration date, sterilization effect of the sterile container.

检查无菌容器的名称、灭菌日期、有效期及灭菌效果。

5. When taking sterile items from a sterile container, take the cover/lid away from the container, keep the inner side of the cover upward on the table or in the hand. Do not touch the edge and the inner surface of a sterile container.

从无菌容器取物时，打开容器盖，盖的内面向上置于台面或拿在手中。手指不可触及无菌容器的边缘及内面。

6. The sterile items should be taken out using sterile transfer forceps.

必须用无菌持物钳/镊从无菌容器内夹取无菌物品。

7. Cover the container immediately after taking out sterile items.

取出无菌物品后，立即将容器盖盖严。

8. When holding a sterile container such as a sterile bowl, hold it from its bottom.

手持无菌容器（如治疗碗）时，应托住容器底部。

New Words and Expressions
单 词 表

conserve [kən'səːv] *vt.* 保存

lid [lid] *n.* 盖子

Nurse Alert 护理事项

1. After removing the lid away from the sterile container, do not let the inner side of the cover downward on the table, and do not expose sterile items inside for a long time.

打开无菌容器后,盖的内面不可向下置于台面,且应避免容器内的无菌物品长时间暴露于空气中。

2. Do not touch the edge and the inner surface of a sterile container.

手指不可触及无菌容器的边缘及内面。

3.3 Applying Sterile Wrapped Packages 无菌包的使用

Purpose 操作目的

Sterile items are wrapped in a variety of sterile materials (muslin/cloth, plastic, etc.) to maintain their sterility for aseptic procedures.

用各种无菌材料(棉布、塑料等)包裹无菌物品以保持物品的无菌状态,供无菌操作使用。

Assessment 评估

1. Assess the working environment to determine whether it is in accordance with the principles of aseptic techniques.

评估操作环境是否符合无菌技术操作原则。

2. Check the name, type, sterilization and expiration date, sterilization effect and integrity of the sterile wrapped package.

检查无菌包的名称、类型、灭菌日期、有效期、灭菌效果及包装的完整性。

Gather equipment 物品准备

Equipments:sterile transfer forceps 无菌持物钳/镊, sterile wrapped package 无菌包, sterile container 无菌容器,sterile field 无菌区,record paper, pen and watch 记录纸、笔和手表。

Procedure 操作过程

1. Report and tidy your dress.

报告并整理仪表。

2. Check the validity of hand sanitizer and wash hands in 7 steps and put on the mask.

检查洗手液的有效期,7 步洗手法洗手并戴口罩。

3. Prepare the equipments. Place equipments on the table in order of use.

准备用物,按使用顺序将用物置于处置桌上。

4. Check the name,type, sterilization and expiration date, sterilization effect and integrity of the sterile package.

检查无菌包的名称、类型、灭菌日期、有效期、灭菌效果及包装的完整性。

5. Check whether the sterile package wrapped in muslin has ever been used and check its shelf life.

检查布类无菌包是否曾开包并检查其保存期限。

6. Open the package.

开包。

(1) Place the sterile package on a clean, dry and flat operating table, untie the string.

将无菌包放在清洁、干燥和平坦的操作台上,解开系带。

(2) Tuck the string and place it under the wrapper of sterile package, grasp the outside surface of the wrapper and open it according to its original creases.

将系带卷放于无菌包的包布下,手持包布外表,按原折叠顺序逐层打开无菌包。

7. Take out sterile items.

取出无菌物品。

(1) Take out a part of sterile items from a sterile package wrapped in muslin.

取出布类无菌包内部分物品。

① Take out items: take out the needed items with a sterile transfer forceps and put them on a prepared sterile container or field.

取物:用无菌持物钳/镊夹取所需物品,放在准备好的无菌容器或无菌区内。

② Fold the package: if the items are remained, fold the sterile package according to its original creases and tie it in a line style.

包扎:如果无菌包内物品未用完,则按原折痕包好,系带横向系紧。

③ Note: note down the date, time of opening the sterile package and your signature.

标记:注明无菌包的开包日期、时间并签名。

④ Post-procedure: replace the sterile package.

整理:将无菌包放回原处。

(2) Taking out all sterile items from a sterile package wrapped in muslin.

取出布类无菌包内全部物品。

① Hold it with one hand, open the wrapper by grasping its four corners with the other hand to expose the items.

一手持无菌包,另一手打开包布并将四角抓住,暴露物品。

② Transfer the items to s sterile container or field or hand to another person who is wearing sterile gloves.

将无菌包内物品放到无菌容器或无菌区内,或传递给另一戴无菌手套的操作者。

New Words and Expressions
单 词 表

muslin [ˈmʌzlin] *n.* 棉布
integrity [inˈtegrəti] *n.* 完整
string [striŋ] *n.* 线,细绳
crease [kriːs] *n.* 折痕;折缝
remain [riˈmein] *vi.* 留下;剩余

Nurse Alert 护理事项

1. When opening a sterile package, do not touch the inside of the wrapper. Do not reach across the sterile field.

打开无菌包时,手不可触及包布的内面,不可跨越无菌区。

2. If the items are expired, contaminated or the wrapper is wet, resterilize them.

如果无菌包内物品超过有效期、被污染或包布潮湿，则需要重新消毒灭菌。

3. Do not use a sterile package when its label is blurred or when it is expired or with leakages or damages.

无菌包如有标签模糊、已过有效期、封包漏气或破损等，均不可使用。

3.4 Preparing a Sterile Tray
铺无菌盘

Purpose 操作目的

To establish a sterile field by placing a sterile drape on a clean and dry tray in order to lay sterile items on it for treatments or nursing care.

将无菌治疗巾铺在清洁、干燥的治疗盘内形成无菌区域，以放置无菌物品，供治疗或护理使用。

Assessment 评估

1. Assess the working environment to determine whether it is in accordance with the principles of aseptic techniques.

评估操作环境是否符合无菌技术操作原则。

2. Check the name, sterilization and expiration date, sterilization effect of the sterile drape.

检查无菌治疗巾的名称、灭菌日期、有效期、灭菌效果等。

Gather equipment 物品准备

Equipments: sterile transfer forceps 无菌持物钳/镊, sterile wrapped package 无菌包, sterile drapes 无菌治疗巾, sterile items 无菌物品, tray 治疗盘, record paper and pen 记录纸和笔。

Procedure 操作过程

1. Report and tidy your dress.

报告并整理仪表。

2. Check the validity of hand sanitizer and wash hands in 7 steps and put on the mask.

检查洗手液的有效期，7 步洗手法洗手并戴口罩。

3. Prepare the equipments. Place equipments on the table in order of use.

准备用物，按使用顺序将用物置于处置桌上。

4. Check the name, sterilization and expiration date, sterilization effect and integrity of the sterile package storing sterile drapes.

检查治疗巾无菌包的名称、灭菌日期、有效期、灭菌效果及包装的完整性。

5. Open the sterile package and take out a sterile drape.

打开无菌包，取出一块无菌治疗巾。

6. Place the sterile drape on a prepared tray.

将无菌治疗巾放在治疗盘内。

7. Lay the sterile drape double layered on the tray, grasp the outer side of two top corners of the sterile drape with both hands and fanfold the edge of the top layer facing outward.

将无菌治疗巾对折铺于治疗盘上，双手捏住无菌治疗巾上层外面两角并折成扇形，边缘向外。

8. Place sterile items on the sterile field as needed.

根据需要将无菌物品放入无菌区内。

9. Pull the top fan-folded layer of the drape to cover the sterile items, fold the end edge of the drape upward twice and then fold the both sides of the edges downward once, leaving the tray edges exposed.

拉开扇形折叠层遮盖于物品上，将开口处向上折两次，两侧边缘分别向下折一次，露出治疗盘边缘。

10. If the prepared sterile tray is not used at once, note down the name, date, time of preparing the sterile tray and your signature.

如果是备用无菌盘，需注明无菌盘的名称、铺盘的日期、时间并签名。

New Words and Expressions
单 词 表

drape [dreip] *n.* 治疗巾

tray [trei] *n.* 托盘;治疗盘

fanfold ['fæn'fəuld] *vt.* 扇形折叠

layer ['leiə] *n.* 层

expose [ik'spəuz] *vt.* 暴露,揭发;使曝光

signature ['signətʃə] *n.* 署名;签名

Nurse Alert 护理事项

1. The surface for preparing a sterile tray should be clean and dry. The sterile drape should not be dampened and contaminated.

铺无菌盘的区域须清洁、干燥,无菌治疗巾应避免潮湿和污染。

2. The prepared sterile tray should be used as soon as possible and its shelf life is up to 4 hours.

铺好的无菌盘应尽早使用,有效期不超过 4 h。

3.5 Pouring Sterile Solutions
取用无菌溶液

Purpose 操作目的

Pour sterile solutions with correct techniques to maintain solutions sterility for aseptic procedures.

正确取用无菌溶液以保持溶液的无菌状态,以供无菌操作使用。

Assessment 评估

1. Assess the working environment to determine whether it is in accordance with

the principles of aseptic techniques.

评估操作环境是否符合无菌技术操作原则。

2. Check the name, concentration, expiration date and quality of sterile solution in a bottle.

检查瓶装无菌溶液的名称、浓度、有效期和质量。

Gather equipment 物品准备

Equipments: tray 治疗盘, sterile solution 无菌溶液, sterile bowl 无菌治疗碗, bottle-top opener 开瓶器, kidney basin 弯盘, antiseptic solution 消毒液, sterile swabs 无菌棉签, sterile forceps 无菌镊子, pen and watch 笔和手表。

Procedure 操作过程

1. Report and tidy your dress.

报告并整理仪表。

2. Check the validity of hand sanitizer and wash hands in 7 steps and put on the mask.

检查洗手液的有效期, 7 步洗手法洗手并戴口罩。

3. Prepare the equipments. Place equipments on the table in order of use.

准备用物, 按使用顺序将用物放置于处置桌上。

4. Obtain a sealed bottle containing sterile solution, clean any dust outside the bottle.

取盛有无菌溶液的密封瓶, 擦净瓶外表灰尘。

5. Check the label (the name of the solution, dosage, concentration and expiration date); check the integrity of the bottle (the bottle cap is not tampered with, and the solution bottle has no chasms); check the quality of sterile solution (the solution is not cloudy, discolored or contains no precipitates).

检查并核对无菌溶液瓶标签(药名、剂量、浓度和有效期); 检查无菌溶液瓶的完好性(瓶盖无松动、瓶身无裂痕); 检查无菌溶液的质量(无浑浊、变色或沉淀)。

6. Remove the aluminium cap with an opener. Check the expiration date of the antiseptic solution, sterile swabs and sterile forceps. Use the sterile forceps to fetch two swabs and dip some sterile solution. Sterilize the surface of the rubber seal. Remove the rubber seal.

用开瓶器撬开瓶盖。检查消毒液、无菌棉签和无菌持物钳/镊的有效期。用无菌持物钳/镊夹取两个无菌棉签并蘸取适量的消毒液。消毒瓶塞表面。拉出瓶塞。

7. With the other hand, hold the bottle with its label in the palm of the hand, pour some solution rotationally to flush the lip of the bottle and then pour solution into a prepared sterile container from the same position.

另一手拿溶液瓶，瓶签朝向掌心，倒出少量溶液旋转冲洗瓶口，再由原处倒出溶液至无菌容器中。

8. On completion, insert the rubber seal into the bottle opening.

倒毕，将瓶塞塞进瓶口。

9. If the solution is remained, note down the date, time of opening and your signature.

如果溶液未用完，需在瓶签上注明开瓶日期、时间并签名。

10. Recheck the label of the bottle, and replace it in correct storage area.

再次核对无菌溶液的标签，将瓶放回原处。

New Words and Expressions

单 词 表

concentration [ˌkɔnsən'treiʃən] *n.* 浓度
bowl [bəul] *n.* 治疗碗
antiseptic [ˌænti'septik] *adj.* 抗菌的
seal [siːl] *n.* 密封
dosage ['dəusidʒ] *n.* 剂量，用量
tamper ['tæmpə] *vi.* 损害
chasm ['kæzəm] *n.* 裂口
precipitate [pri'sipiteit] *n.* [化学] 沉淀物
aluminium [ˌæljuː'miniəm] *adj.* 铝的 *n.* 铝
palm [pɑːm] *n.* 手掌
rotationally [rəu'teiʃənəli] *adv.* 旋转地
flush [flʌʃ] *vt.* 用水冲洗
completion [kəm'pliːʃən] *n.* 完成，结束

Nurse Alert 护理事项

1. Do not dip the sterile solution in a bottle directly.

不可直接将物品伸入无菌溶液瓶内蘸取溶液。

2. Before pouring sterile solutions, pour a small amount of solution to clean the lip of the bottle.

倒无菌溶液前,先倒出少量溶液冲洗瓶口。

3. Once the solution is poured, do not return it in order to avoid contaminating the remained solution. The remained sterile solution in the bottle needs to be used within 24 hours.

已倒出的溶液不可再倒回瓶内以免污染剩余的溶液,瓶内剩余的无菌溶液限 24 h 内使用。

3.6 Donning and Removing Sterile Gloves
戴、摘无菌手套

Purpose 操作目的

When performing aseptic procedures, donning and removing sterile gloves with correct techniques can maintain the sterility effect during procedures and protect patients and health care workers against infections.

在进行无菌操作时,正确戴、摘无菌手套可以确保操作的无菌效果及保护患者及医务人员免受感染。

Assessment 评估

1. Assess the working environment to determine whether it is in accordance with the principles of aseptic techniques.

评估操作环境是否符合无菌技术操作原则。

2. Check the type, size, sterilization/manufacture and expiration date, sterilization effect of the sterile gloves.

检查无菌手套的类型、号码、灭菌/生产日期、有效期及灭菌效果。

Gather equipment 物品准备

sterile disposable gloves 一次性无菌手套
kidney basin 弯盘
medical waste bag 医用垃圾袋

Procedure 操作过程

1. Choose a pair of sterile gloves of appropriate size for yourself.

选择号码合适的无菌手套。

2. Check the type, sterilization/manufacture and expiration date, sterilization effect of sterile gloves and the integrity of its package.

检查无菌手套的类型、灭菌/生产日期、有效期、灭菌效果及包装的完整性。

3. Open the package of sterile gloves.

打开无菌手套袋。

(1) Open the outer package, and then take out the inner package.

打开外包装,取出内包装。

(2) Place the inner package on a clean and dry operating table or a sterile field, carefully open the inner package according to its original creases so that the cuffs of the sterile gloves are closest to you.

将内包装放于清洁、干燥的操作台上或无菌区内,按原折叠顺序逐层打开内包装,并使手套的袖口端靠近操作者。

(3) Take out the packet of powder and apply it to hands if necessary.

必要时取出滑石粉包擦涂双手。

4. Put on sterile gloves.

戴无菌手套。

(1) Picking up gloves one by one. 分次取手套法。

① With one hand, grasp the folded cuff edge of the glove (the glove's inside surface), lift it up and away from the wrapper; carefully pull the glove over the other hand.

一手捏住一只手套的袖口反折部分(手套内面),取出手套,并对准另一只手戴上。

② With your gloved hand, slip your finger underneath the second glove's cuff (the glove's outside surface), lift it up and away from the wrapper; carefully pull the second glove over your second hand using the same method.

用戴好手套的手指插入另一只手套的袖口反折内面(手套外面),取出手套,同法戴好第二只手的手套。

(2) Picking up gloves together. 一次性取手套法。

① With your hands, grasp the folded edge of cuff of each glove respectively (the glove's inside surface), lift them up and away from the wrapper.

两只手分别捏住两只手套的袖口反折处(手套内面),取出手套。

② Pull the first glove over your first hand; with your gloved hand, slip your finger underneath the second glove's cuff (the glove's outside surface), pull the second glove over your second hand using the same method.

将手套五指对准,先戴一只手套;再以戴好手套的手指插入另一只手套的袖口反折内面(手套外面),同法戴好。

③ Adjust each glove so that it fits smoothly, and unfold the cuffs down over your uniform sleeves.

用双手将手套位置调整平顺,将手套的翻边扣套在工作服衣袖外面。

④ Remove the powder on the outer glove surface by rinsing the gloved hands with sterile water as needed before performing aseptic procedures.

在无菌操作前,按需用无菌水冲洗干净手套表面的滑石粉。

⑤ With one gloved hand, pinch up the outside surface of the glove for the other hand at the wrist and pull it off so that the glove inverts itself, with the contaminated surface inside.

用戴手套的一只手捏住另一只手的手套腕部外面,翻转摘下,使污染面在内。

⑥ Slip one finger of the bare hand into the wrist under the cuff of the other glove and pull the second glove off, inverting it over itself.

将脱下手套的手指插入另一手套内,将其翻转摘下。

⑦ Discard the used gloves in a kidney basin or medical waste bag.

将用过的手套放入弯盘或医用垃圾袋内。

⑧ Wash hands thoroughly.

洗手。

New Words and Expressions

单 词 表

cuff [kʌf] *n.* 袖口

wrapper [ˈræpə] *n.* 包装材料；[包装] 包装纸

respectively [riˈspektivli] *adv.* 分别地；各自地

rinse [rins] *vt.* 漱；冲洗掉

pinch [pintʃ] *vt.* 捏

invert [inˈvəːt] *vt.* 使……颠倒；使……反转

bare [bɛə] *adj.* 空的；赤裸的

Nurse Alert 护理事项

1. When putting on sterile gloves, your bare hands can not touch the outside of the gloves, the gloved hand can not touch the other bare hand or the inside of the other glove.

戴无菌手套时，未戴手套的手不可触及手套的外面，已经戴好手套的手不可触及未戴手套的手及另一手套的内面。

2. After putting on sterile gloves, keep hands from the waist or the level of operating table to eye level. If the glove is punctured, contaminated or contaminated in doubt, remove the glove or put on a new glove over it immediately.

戴上无菌手套后，只能接触无菌物品，双手始终保持在腰部或操作台面以上、视线范围以内。手套如有破洞、污染或可疑污染，应立即更换或加戴无菌手套。

Communication Model
沟通模板

Self-introduction Model 常规介绍模板

Good morning/afternoon teachers, my name is ××, I come from class ××, my student's number is ××. Today, I am going to show you the process of aseptic technique, the equipments I have prepared are..., everything is ready, may I start?

老师早上好/下午好，我的名字是××，来自××班，我的学号是××。今天我要展示的操作是无菌技术，所准备的用物有……，准备完毕，请求开始。

Assessment 评估

1. The working environment is clean with adequate space and lighting.

操作环境清洁、宽敞、明亮。

2. The operating table is clean, dry and flat.

操作台面清洁、干燥、平坦。

3. There was no cleaning half an hour ago.

半小时内无人打扫。

Communication 沟通

1. Check the tray: the tray is clean and dry. It can be used.

治疗盘检查:治疗盘清洁干燥,可以使用。

2. Check the sterile forceps: sterile forceps. Sterilization date: ××. In the effective range. It can be used. (The same as the sterile swabs and sterile storage tank.)

检查无菌持物钳/镊:无菌持物钳/镊。灭菌日期:××。在有效期范围内。可以使用。(无菌棉签及无菌储槽的检查同无菌持物钳/镊。)

3. Check the sterile package: sterile drapes. Sterilization date: ××. In the effective range. Indicator tape has turned into black. No moist and damage. It can be used.

检查无菌包:无菌治疗巾。灭菌日期:××。在有效期范围内。指示胶带变为黑色。无潮湿和破损。可以使用。

4. Check the sterile solution: normal saline. Dosage: 250 milliliter. Concentration: 0.9%. Expiration date: ××. In the effective range. The bottle cap is not tampered with and the solution bottle has no chasms, the solution is not cloudy, discolored or contains no particle or precipitates. It can be used.

检查无菌溶液:生理盐水。剂量:250 mL。浓度:0.9%。有效期:××。在有效期范围内。瓶盖无松动,瓶身无裂痕,溶液无浑浊、无变色、无杂质及沉淀物。可以使用。

Scoring Criteria 5
评分细则 5

项目		总分	技术操作要求	标准分	扣分说明	扣分
评估 10	仪表	2	仪表端庄、服装整洁、修剪指甲、洗手、戴口罩	2	一项不符扣 2 分	
	环境	4	环境清洁、宽敞，30 min 内无打扫	2	一项不符扣 1 分	
			操作台清洁、干燥、平坦	2	一项不符扣 1 分	
	物品	4	用物齐备，物品摆放位置恰当	2	一项不符扣 1 分	
			检查无菌物品有效期	2	一项不符扣 1 分	
实施 70	无菌包的使用	15	检查无菌包标签（名称、有效期、灭菌指示带、有无潮湿和破损）	4	一项不符扣 1 分	
			开包方法正确（由外向内依序开包，包带不松散，未碰内侧面）	4	一项不符扣 2 分	
			取物方法正确，未跨越无菌区，无污染（使用卵圆钳）	3	一项不符扣 1 分	
			用毕包扎方法正确（原折痕包好，系带横向扎好，标明时间及开包者姓名）	4	一项不符扣 1 分	
	无菌钳的使用	15	检查有效期，持钳方法正确	3	一项不符扣 1 分	
			取钳方法正确（不触及筒内壁边缘，筒盖及时关闭）	4	一项不符扣 2 分	
			使用方法正确（钳端向下，不倒转）	4	一项不符扣 2 分	
			放钳方法正确（不触及筒内壁，盖盖，打开轴节）	4	一项不符扣 2 分	
	铺无菌盘及取无菌溶液	40	治疗盘清洁干燥	1	一项不符扣 1 分	
			铺无菌巾方法正确（单层）	2	一项不符扣 2 分	
			扇形折叠正确（边缘向外）	2	一项不符扣 2 分	
			一次性取出无菌包内物品正确	4	一项不符扣 2 分	
			擦净药瓶	1	一项不符扣 1 分	
			检查药液并核对（药名、剂量、浓度、有效期，瓶盖无松动，瓶身无裂痕，药液无沉淀、浑浊、絮状物及变色）	6	一项不符扣 1 分	
			检查无菌棉签有效期，取无菌棉签方法正确	4	一项不符扣 2 分	
			检查消毒液有效期，消毒瓶口方法正确（两次方向相反，公转并自转）；开启瓶盖	4	一项不符扣 2 分	
			持液体瓶（标签向掌心）、冲瓶口、倒液方法正确	3	一项不符扣 1 分	
			标明无菌液体开瓶时间及姓名	2	一项不符扣 1 分	
			检查无菌储槽有效期	1	一项不符扣 1 分	
			开储槽方法正确，取物正确，无污染	2	一项不符扣 2 分	
			无菌盘物品放置合理	2	一项不符扣 2 分	
			无菌盘覆盖边缘折叠整齐（开口处向上折两次，两边向下折叠一次）	3	一项不符扣 1 分	
			无菌盘标明名称、时间及姓名	3	一项不符扣 1 分	

续表

项　目		总分	技术操作要求	标准分	扣分说明	扣分
评价 20	熟练	4	操作轻稳、熟练，步骤合理	4	一项不符扣1分	
	效果	6	无菌观念强、操作过程无污染	6	一项不符扣3分	
	英语	10	发音准确，语言流畅、熟练	10	酌情扣分	
主考教师签字：			日期：	总分：100	得分：	

评分标准：91～100分为优，81～90分为良，71～80分为中，60～70分为差，低于60分为不及格。

注：跨越无菌区3～5次，或污染不多于2次，得分不超过80分；跨越无菌区多于5次或污染不少于3次，考核为不及格。

Chapter 4
Isolation Technique
隔离技术

4.1 Hand Washing
洗　　手

Purpose 操作目的

Hand washing can ensure that all skin surfaces are thoroughly cleaned in order to remove all soil and a major part of transient microorganisms on hands.

洗手能使手部皮肤得到彻底清洁，去除手部污垢和大部分暂居菌。

Assessment 评估

1. Determine the method of hand washing that is most appropriate for assigned task.

确定最合适的洗手方法。

2. Assess the availability of equipment for hand washing.

评估有无洗手设备。

Gather equipment 物品准备

hand washing pool with non-manual switch 非手动开关洗手池，

running water 流动水，

soap or liquid soap 肥皂或皂液，

Automatic hand dryer, paper towels or dry towels 感应式干手机、纸巾或干毛巾。

Procedure　操作过程

1. Remove any rings, jewelry and wristwatch. Roll the sleeves 10-20 cm above the wrist. Ensure that the nails are clipped short.

取下手上饰物、手表，衣袖上推到腕上 10～20 cm，剪短指甲。

2. Check hands and fingers for cuts or abrasions, any cuts or abrasions on the hands should be covered with a waterproof, occlusive dressing.

检查手上有无伤口，任何伤口都应先贴好防水敷贴。

3. Stand in front of the sink. Do not allow your clothing to touch the sink during the washing procedure.

站在洗手池前，洗手过程中衣服不要触及洗手池。

4. Turn on water using non-manual switch so that the flow is adequate, but not splashing.

采用非手动开关打开流动水，使水量充足但不会溅出。

5. Wet the hands and wrist area under running water. Keep hands lower than elbows to allow water toward fingertips.

用流动水打湿双手和手腕。保持手的位置低于肘部，使水流向指尖。

6. Place an appropriate amount of soap or liquid soap on hands and thoroughly distribute over hands.

取适量肥皂或皂液，均匀涂抹于双手。

7. Use firm and circular motions to rub the hands for minimum of 15 seconds, covering all areas including the palms, backs of the hands, fingers, the areas between the fingers, knuckles, fingertips and wrists. The seven-step hand washing technique is recommended.

认真揉搓双手至少 15 s。揉搓双手的每个部位，包括手掌、手背、手指、指缝、指关节、指尖和手腕。推荐采用 7 步洗手法。

(1) Palm to palm with fingers closed and rub together.

掌心对掌心，手指并拢相互揉搓。

(2) One palm over the back of the other hand with fingers interlaced and rub between fingers, and vice versa.

掌心对手背，手指交叉沿指缝相互揉搓，两手交替。

(3) Palm to palm with fingers interlaced and rub between fingers.

掌心对掌心，手指交叉沿指缝相互揉搓。

(4) Backs of fingers to opposing palms with fingers interlocked and rub together.

两手互握，互搓指背。

(5) Rotational rubbing of one thumb clasped in the other palm, and vice versa.

一只手握另一只手拇指旋转揉搓，两手交替。

(6) Rotational rubbing, forwards and backwards with clasped fingertips of one hand in the other palm, and vice versa.

指尖在掌心中旋转揉搓，两手交替。

(7) If necessary, rotational rubbing of one wrist in the other hand, and vice versa.

必要时握住手腕，旋转揉搓，两手交替。

8. Rinse your hands thoroughly under running water, keeping fingers pointed downward until all traces of soap are removed.

在流动水下彻底冲净双手，指尖朝下，直至皂液冲净为止。

9. Resoap your hands, rewash, and rerinse if heavily contaminated.

如果手污染严重，重新取用肥皂/皂液，再次揉搓并清洗。

10. Turn off the tap with your foot or elbow. If the tap is not elbow-or foot-operated or automatically controlled, leave the water running until after drying your hands and then use a paper towel to turn off the tap.

用脚踏或手肘关水龙头。如果水龙头不是肘动、脚踏或感应式开关，应先擦干双手再用纸巾关水龙头。

11. Dry your hands thoroughly with a paper towel, or an automatic hand dryer. If using clean towels to dry, disinfect the towel after one time use.

用纸巾擦干双手，或用感应式干手机吹干双手。如果使用清洁毛巾擦干手，毛巾应一用一消毒。

New Words and Expressions
单 词 表

soil [sɔil] *n.* 污垢

transient [ˈtrænziənt] *adj.* 短暂的

microorganism [ˌmaikrəuˈɔːgəˌnizəm] *n.* [微]微生物

clip [klip] *vt*. 修剪
abrasion [ə'breiʒən] *n*. 擦伤
occlusive [ə'klu:siv] *adj*. 闭塞的 ;密封的
splash [splæʃ] *vt*. 溅,泼
knuckle ['nʌkl] *n*. 关节;指关节
vice versa 反之亦然
interlace [ˌintə'leis] *vt*. 使交错,使交织
interlock [ˌintə'lɔk] *v*. 使联结
thumb [θʌm] *n*. 拇指
rotational [rau'teiʃənl] *adj*. 转动的;回转的;轮流的
trace [treis] *n*. 痕迹,踪迹

4.2 Donning and Removing an Isolation Gown 穿、脱隔离衣

Purpose 操作目的

1. To protect health care workers and patients.
保护医务人员和患者。
2. To prevent the spread of microorganisms in order to avoid cross-infection.
防止病原微生物撒播,避免交叉感染。

Assessment 评估

1. Assess the patient's health condition, the type of isolation and isolation measures.
评估患者病情、采取的隔离种类及隔离措施。
2. Assess the purpose of entering the patient's isolation room and all necessary equipment.
评估本次进入患者隔离单位的目的和需要的用物。
3. Assess the working environment and apparatus for hand washing and hand antisepsis.
评估操作环境、洗手及手消毒的设施。

Gather equipment 物品准备

isolation gown 隔离衣

sterile disposable gloves 一次性无菌手套

apparatus for hand washing and hand antisepsis 洗手及手消毒设施

Procedure 操作过程

1. Report and tidy your dress.

报告并整理仪表。

2. Wash hands in 7 steps and put on the headgear and mask.

7 步洗手法洗手，戴帽子及口罩。

3. Select an isolation gown of appropriate type and size for yourself. Take an isolation gown by holding its collar so that the inside is toward you. Fold the two sides of the collar in order to expose the armholes of the sleeves.

选择种类及号码合适的隔离衣。手持衣领取隔离衣，清洁面朝向操作者。将衣领两端向外折。露出肩袖内口。

4. Hold the collar with one hand, slip the other hand into the sleeve, and raise the arm to pull the sleeve up. Put on the other sleeve using the same method.

一只手持衣领，另一只手伸入衣袖内，举起手臂，将衣袖穿好。同法穿好另一只袖。

5. Hold the collar and move the hands from the center of the collar to the two ends, button up or tie strings at your back of neck.

两手持衣领，由前向后理顺领边，在颈后扣上领扣或系好衣领。

6. Wrap the gown around your wrist, button up or tie stings around your wrist, use a rubber band to tie it as needed.

卷紧袖口，扣好袖口或系上袖带，需要时用橡皮圈束紧袖口。

7. Grasp one side of the gown about 5 cm below waist level, pull it forward, reach and pinch the edge, reach and pinch the other edge of the gown using the same method.

自一侧衣缝腰带下 5 cm 处将隔离衣向前拉至衣边处捏住，同法将另一侧一边捏住。

8. Align the gown edges at your back, overlap the gown toward one side of your back and press the folded part.

两手在背后将衣边边缘对齐，向一边折叠并按住折叠处。

9. Cross the strings on your back, turn them to your front and make a free tie.

将腰带在背后交叉，回到身体的前面打活结系好。

10. Put on the sterile gloves.

戴无菌手套。

11. Take off the gloves. Untie waist strings and make a free tie in the front of the gown.

脱下手套。解开腰带，在前面打活结。

12. Unbutton or untie the cuffs of the sleeves, tuck part of the gown sleeves on the elbow uniform sleeves.

解开袖口，在肘部将部分衣袖塞入工作衣袖内。

13. Disinfect your hands using the method according to local policy.

按当地要求的方法消毒双手。

14. Unbutton or untie neck stings.

解开领口。

15. Insert the right hand into the inside of the left sleeve at wrist, pull sleeve wristlet over the left hand.

右手伸入左手袖口内，拉下衣袖使其遮住左手。

16. Use your left gown-covered hand to pull the outside part of sleeve wristlet over your right hand. Working from the inside of the gown, side the gown down the arms and pull sleeves off your arms.

再用衣袖遮住的左手在外面拉下右手衣袖。双手在袖内将衣袖拉下使双臂退出。

17. If the isolation gown will be reused, hold the gown with both hands at the inside shoulder seams. Bring the hands together, invert one shoulder over the other so that the clean inside surface is outermost. Align the collar and two sides of gown and then hang it on a hook.

若隔离衣需重复使用，双手撑着隔离衣内面双肩接缝处。双手并拢，将一侧隔离衣肩部反折至另一侧上，使隔离衣清洁面（内面）朝外。将隔离衣衣领及其两边对齐后挂在衣钩上。

18. If the gown will not be reused, fold the gown up inside out and discard it into the linen hamper for the soiled linen (or according to local policy).

不再穿的隔离衣，将清洁面（内面）朝外卷好放入污衣袋内（或按当地要求）。

19. Wash hands.

洗手。

20. Remove the mask.

摘口罩。

New Words and Expressions
单 词 表

apparatus [ˌæpəˈreitəs] *n.* 装置,设备

gown [gaun] *n.* 长袍

string [striŋ] *n.* 线,细绳

pinch [pintʃ] *vt.* 捏

align [əˈlain] *vt.* 使结盟;使成一行;匹配

overlap [ˌəuvəˈlæp] *n.* 重叠

wristlet [ˈristlit] *n.* 腕套

seam [siːm] *n.* 缝;接缝

outermost [ˈautəˌməʊst] *adj.* 最外面的

Nurse Alert 护理事项

1. When donning and removing an isolation gown, do not contaminate the collar and the clean side and keep the collar clean all the time.

穿、脱隔离衣过程中避免污染衣领和清洁面,始终保持衣领清洁。

2. After wearing an isolation gown, keep arms from the waist to eye level. Do not go into the clean area to avoid touching clean items.

穿好隔离衣后,双臂保持在腰部以上、视线范围以内,不得进入清洁区,避免接触清洁物品。

3. While disinfecting hands, do not wet the gown and do not allow the gown to touch the surrounding items.

消毒手时不能沾湿隔离衣,隔离衣也不可触及其他物品。

4. Change isolation gowns daily or according to local policy. If a gown is dampened or contaminated, replace it immediately.

隔离衣每日更换或按当地要求操作,如有潮湿或污染,应立即更换。

5. When hanging an isolation gown, the clean inside surface is outermost in half-contaminated area, he contaminated outside surface is outermost in contaminated area.

挂在半污染区的隔离衣清洁面向外,挂在污染区的则污染面向外。

Communication Model
沟通模板

Self-introduction Model 常规介绍模板

Good morning/afternoon teachers, my name is ××, I come from class ××, my student's number is ××. Today, I am going to show you the process of isolation technique, the equipments I have prepared are..., everything is ready, may I start?

老师早上好/下午好,我是××,来自××班,我的学号为××。我今天做的操作是隔离技术,所需用物有……,用物准备齐全,请求开始。

Assessment 评估

1. The working environment is clean with adequate space.

操作环境清洁,适宜操作。

2. The isolation gown is not moist and damaged.

隔离衣清洁干燥,无破损。

Scoring Criteria 6
评分细则 6

项目		总分	技术操作要求	标准分	扣分说明	得分
评估 10	仪表	2	仪表端庄、服装整洁、修剪指甲、洗手（取下手表、衣袖卷至肘上）、戴口罩	2	一项不符扣 2 分	
	环境	4	环境整洁、宽敞	2	一项不符扣 1 分	
			明确患者隔离的种类	2	一项不符扣 2 分	
	物品	4	检查隔离衣（无潮湿、破损）	2	一项不符扣 1 分	
			物品齐备	2	一项不符扣 2 分	
实施 70	穿隔离衣	25	提衣领，取下隔离衣，清洁面朝向自己	2	一项不符扣 1 分	
			穿衣袖方法正确（不触及外侧面）	4	一项不符扣 1 分	
			系衣领扣手法正确（下颌、面部不触及隔离衣）	4	一项不符扣 2 分	
			扎袖口方法正确（手不可触及隔离衣内面）	4	一项不符扣 2 分	
			系腰带方法正确，不触及内侧面	4	一项不符扣 2 分	
			腰带下 5 cm 处，后襟对齐，向一侧折叠	3	一项不符扣 1 分	
			腰带在背后交叉，回到前面打结	4	一项不符扣 2 分	
	戴脱手套	15	核对（手套号码、有效期）	2	一项不符扣 1 分	
			取手套方法正确、不污染	2	一项不符扣 2 分	
			戴手套方法正确、不污染	8	一项不符扣 2 分	
			脱手套方法正确、不污染	2	一项不符扣 1 分	
			手套置于医用垃圾桶内	1	一项不符扣 1 分	
	刷手及脱隔离衣	30	解腰带在前方打一活结	2	一项不符扣 2 分	
			解袖口，挽袖口方法正确（不接触内侧面）	4	一项不符扣 2 分	
			消毒手范围、顺序、方法正确	6	一项不符扣 2 分	
			消毒手时间充分	2	一项不符扣 2 分	
			消毒手过程中不污染隔离衣	2	一项不符扣 2 分	
			擦手方法正确	2	一项不符扣 1 分	
			脱隔离衣方法、步骤正确	6	一项不符扣 2 分	
			不污染工作服	2	一项不符扣 2 分	
			挂隔离衣方法正确	2	一项不符扣 2 分	
			取下口罩正确（污染面向内折叠，不接触污染面）	2	一项不符扣 2 分	
评价 20	熟练	6	操作轻稳、熟练、步骤合理	4	一项不符扣 2 分	
			按规定时间完成（穿脱时间 6 min）	2	每超过 30 s 扣 1 分	
	效果	4	隔离概念明确、无污染	4	酌情扣分	
	英文	10	发音准确，语言流畅、熟练	10	酌情扣分	
主考教师：			日期：	总分：100	得分：	

评分标准：91～100 分为优，81～90 分为良，71～80 分为中，60～70 分为差，低于 60 分为不及格。

注：1. 未刷手即脱隔离衣，该项考核为不及格。

2. 隔离观念不明确，污染≤3 次，得分不超过 80 分；污染≥5 次，该项考核为不及格。

Chapter 5
Assessing Vital Signs
生命体征的评估

5.1 Measuring Body Temperature
体温的测量

Purpose 操作目的

1. To determine whether the patient's body temperature is within normal range.

判断患者的体温是否正常。

2. To monitor the changes of body temperature dynamically in order to analyze the patient's heat pattern.

动态监测体温的变化，以分析患者的热型。

3. To aid in the diagnosis or to provide data for disease prevention, treatments, rehabilitation and nursing care.

协助诊断或为预防、治疗、康复和护理提供依据。

Assessment 评估

1. Assess the patient's age, level of consciousness, health condition, psychological status and ability to cooperate.

评估患者的年龄、意识、病情、心理状态及配合程度。

2. Assess factors that can alter the patient is body temperature such as exercising,

eating, drinking cold or hot liquids, receiving heat or cold therapy, bathing or performing hipbath, administering enema.

评估有无影响患者体温变化的因素,如运动、进食、冷热饮、接受冷疗或热疗法、洗澡或沐浴、灌肠等。

3. Assess the condition of the patient is oral mucous membranes, the axillary or anus skin for obtaining body temperature. Determine the most appropriate site to obtain body temperature.

评估患者测量体温的部位(口腔黏膜、腋窝及肛门皮肤)的状况,确定最适合的体温测量部位。

Gather equipment 物品准备

tray 治疗盘, curved basin 弯盘, gauze or tissues 纱布或纸巾, mercury thermometer 水银体温计, record chart and pen 记录单和笔, a watch with a second hand 表(有秒针), lubricant 润滑剂, swabs 棉签, tissues and disposable gloves (for taking a rectal temperature) 纸巾和一次性手套(用于测量肛温), hand sanitizer 洗手液。

Procedure 操作过程

1. Report and tidy your dress.

报告并整理仪表。

2. Check the validity of hand sanitizer and wash hands in 7 steps and put on the mask.

检查洗手液的有效期,7 步洗手法洗手并戴口罩。

3. Prepare the equipments. Check the quality of the thermometer and whether the temperature reading on the thermometer is below 35 ℃. If necessary, shake the mercury thermometer to lower mercury level.

准备用物。检查体温计的质量及读数是否在 35 ℃以下。必要时,将体温计的水银柱甩下。

4. Wash hands and remove the mask.

洗手、摘口罩。

5. Take the equipment to the bedside. Evaluate the environment of the ward.

携用物到患者床边。评估病室环境是否适宜操作。

6. Check the patient's bed number and name. Explain the purpose for the

operation.

核对患者床号与姓名。解释操作目的。

7. Assess the patient to comfortable position.

协助患者取舒适体位。

8. Take body temperature using an appropriate method and tell the patient the precautions.

选用适当的方法测量体温并告知患者注意事项。

(1) Taking an oral temperature 口温测量法

① Assist the patient to comfortable position.

协助患者取舒适体位。

② Ask the patient to open his/her mouth, and place the bulb of the oral thermometer in sublingual heat pocket. Ask the patient to close the lips but not to bite on the thermometer. Leave the thermometer in place for 3 minutes.

嘱患者张口,将口表水银端放于舌下热窝处。指导患者闭紧口唇但勿咬体温计。放置时间为 3 min。

(2) Taking an axillary temperature 腋温测量法

① Assist the patient to comfortable position.

协助患者取舒适体位。

② Expose the patient's axilla. If the axilla is moist, dry it with a towel or tissues.

暴露患者腋窝。如果有汗,用毛巾或纸巾擦干。

③ Place the bulb of the axillary thermometer in the center of axilla. Assist the patient to flex the arm across the chest to secure the thermometer. Leave the thermometer in place for 10 minutes.

将腋表水银端置于腋窝中央。协助患者屈臂过胸以夹紧体温计。放置时间为 10 min。

(3) Taking a rectal temperature 肛温测量法

① Ensure the patient's privacy by drawing screens.

屏风遮挡以保护患者的隐私。

② Wear disposable gloves. Assist the patient to comfortable position: lying on side, abdomen, or back with knees slightly flexed, leaving only the buttocks exposed.

戴一次性手套。协助患者取舒适体位:侧卧位、俯卧位或屈膝仰卧位,只暴露臀部。

③ Lubricate the bulb of the rectal thermometer.

润滑肛表水银端。

④ Separate the patient's buttocks with one hand to expose anus. Instruct the patient to relax by taking deep breaths. With the other hand, gently insert the bulb of the rectal thermometer into the anus and fix it. The length of insertion varies according to the patient's age:3-4 cm for adults, 2 cm for children, 1.25 cm for infants. Leave the thermometer in place for 3 minutes.

一只手分开臀部,暴露患者肛门。指导患者深呼吸放松。另一只手轻轻将肛表插入其肛门并固定。插入深度视患者的年龄而定:成人 3～4 cm，小儿 2 cm，婴幼儿 1.25 cm。体温计放置时间为 3 min。

9. Remove the thermometer and wipe it with tissues and discard the tissues.

取出体温计,用纸巾擦净体温计并弃去纸巾。

10. After taking a rectal temperature, clean the anus and assist the patient to put on pants.

测量肛温结束,擦净肛门并协助患者穿好裤子。

11. Hold the thermometer at eye level, avoid touching the bulb of the thermometer. Rotate the thermometer until the mercury column is clearly visible, read the temperature and inform the patient of temperature reading.

手持体温计与视线平行,注意勿接触体温计水银端。转动体温计至能看清水银柱,读取体温值并告知患者。

12. Place the thermometer on the gauze in a curved basin.

将体温计放于弯盘内纱布上。

13. Record the body temperature reading.

记录体温值。

14. Explain the importance of monitoring body temperature, instruct the correct techniques of taking body temperature and tell the related precautions to patient in order to obtain an accurate temperature reading.

向患者解释体温监测的重要性,指导患者测量体温的正确方法,告知患者测量体温过程中的注意事项,以获取准确的体温值。

15. Inform the patient of the normal range of body temperature. If hyperthermia or hyperthermia occurs, provide related education according to his/her health condition.

向患者介绍正常的体温值范围。如果体温过高或过低,则根据患者病情提供相关的指导。

16. Assist the patient to comfortable position and tidy up clothing.

协助患者取舒适体位,整理衣物。

17. Ask the patient's feelings and needs.

询问患者的感受及需求。

18. Tidy up the patient's bed.

整理床单位。

19. Discard all used equipment appropriately.

合理清理用物。

20. Disinfect the thermometer and store it appropriately.

正确消毒体温计并存放。

21. Wash hands.

洗手。

22. Sign the treatment sheet or nursing care plan to indicate that the body temperature has been taken.

在治疗单或护理计划单上签名，表示已测量体温。

23. Record the body temperature on the vital sign flowsheet or nursing record according to local policy.

按当地要求绘制体温单或在护理记录单上记录。

Nurse Alert　护理事项

1. Before assessing a patient's body temperature, check the quality of the thermometer and read the mercury level to see whether it is below 35 ℃. If assessing temperature for many patients in the same time, count the thermometers before and after assessing to avoid lost or breakage of the thermometers.

测量体温前，应检查体温计的质量及水银柱是否在 35 ℃以下。集体测温时，测温前后应清点体温计的数量，以防丢失或打破体温计。

2. Note factors that can alter the patient's body temperature. Wait 30 minutes before taking body temperature if the patient has been exercising, eating, drinking cold or hot liquids, receiving heat or cold therapy, bathing, performing hipbath or administering enema.

注意评估有无影响患者体温变化的因素。若有运动、进食、冷热饮、冷热疗、洗澡、坐浴或灌肠等，应等待 30 min 后测量。

3. Select the most appropriate site for obtaining body temperature. The neck or groin is used to take body temperature for infants.

选择患者最合适的测量体温的部位。婴幼儿可采用颈部或腹股沟测量。

(1) Oral method is only used for alert and cooperative patients, and is not appropriate for infants, "mouth breathers", patients who are confused or unconscious, have oral disease or have undergone oral surgery.

口温测量法仅适用于清醒、合作的患者，婴幼儿、张口呼吸者、精神异常、昏迷、口腔疾患及口腔手术的患者忌用口温测量法。

(2) Axillary method is safe but time-consuming. It is not appropriate for patients who have axilla surgery or with severely sweating in axilla, with injured shoulder joint or severely thin patients.

腋温测量法安全但耗时。腋下有创伤、炎症、手术和腋下出汗较多者，以及肩关节受伤或过于消瘦的患者忌用腋温测量法。

(3) Rectal method is contraindicated for patients who have undergone rectal or anus surgery, or have diarrhea or acute myocardial infarction.

直肠或肛门手术、腹泻及急性心肌梗死患者忌用肛温测量法。

4. Use mercury thermometer safely.

安全使用水银体温计。

(1) If the patient is very young, severely ill or restless, arrange a person to remain with the patient and hold the thermometer in place.

对婴幼儿、危重或躁动的患者，应配备专人看护并固定好体温计。

(2) If a patient accidentally bites the thermometer and breaks it, remove the glasses from the mouth immediately, and then let the patient consume egg white or milk to postpone the absorption of mercury. If permitted, consume food with crude fiber to promote its elimination.

若患者不慎咬破体温计，首先立即清理玻璃碎屑，再让患者口服蛋清或牛奶以延缓对汞的吸收。如果病情允许，可进食粗纤维食物，加速汞的排出。

5. Arrange the care plan for taking temperature according to the patient's health condition.

根据病情制订测量体温的计划。

(1) For a newly admitted patient, take temperature 4 times per day for 3 days, and then 2 times per day when the temperature is within normal range or according to local policy.

新入院患者：每日测量体温 4 次，连续测量 3 天，3 天后体温正常者改为每天测量 2 次或按当地要求测量。

(2) For a surgical patient, take temperature 4 times per day for the day before operation and 3 days after operation, and then 2 times per day when the temperature is

within normal range or according to local policy.

手术患者:手术前1天及手术后3天内每天测量体温4次,体温恢复正常后改为每天测量2次或按当地要求测量。

(3) Observe temperature changes closely for patients who are severely ill, with hyperthermia or hypothermia and premature babies. Recheck the temperature 30 minutes after temperature-lowering interventions.

危重患者、高热或体温过低患者、早产儿需严密观察体温变化。采用降温措施后30 min应复测体温。

6. If the temperature reading does not correspond to the patient's condition, reassess the temperature. If the temperature is abnormal, observe his/her symptoms and signs, and report to the doctor.

体温与病情不相符时,应重新测量。体温异常者,应观察其伴随症状、体征,并向医生汇报。

New Words and Expressions
单 词 表

dynamically [daiˈnæmikəli] *adv.* 动态地
analyze [ˈænəlaiz] *vt.* 对……进行分析,分解
administering [ədˈministəriŋ] *v.* 管理;实施
mercury [ˈməːkjuri] *n.* 水银
monitoring [ˈmɔnitəriŋ] *n.* 检验,检查
hyperthermia [ˌhaipəˈθəːmiə] *n.* 过高热
flowsheet [fləuˈʃiːt] *n.* 程序框图

5.2 Assessing Pulse
脉搏的测量

Purpose 操作目的

1. To determine whether the patient's pulse is within normal range.

判断患者的脉搏是否正常。

2. To monitor the changes of pulse dynamically in order to assess the patient's cardiac status indirectly.

动态监测脉搏的变化，间接了解患者的心脏状况。

3. To aid in the diagnosis or to provide data for disease prevention, treatments, rehabilitation and nursing care.

协助诊断或为预防、治疗、康复和护理提供依据。

Assessment 评估

1. Assess the patient's age, level of consciousness, health condition, treatments, medications, psychological status and ability to cooperate.

评估患者的年龄、意识、病情、治疗、用药、心理状态及配合程度。

2. Assess factors that can alter the pulse rate, such as acute exercising, stress, fear or crying.

评估有无影响患者脉率变化的因素，如剧烈运动、紧张、恐惧、哭闹等。

3. Assess the skin on the site for assessing pulse and select an appropriate site to obtain pulse.

评估测量脉搏部位的皮肤情况并选择适合的测量部位。

Gather equipment 物品准备

a watch with a second hand 表(有秒针), record chart and pen 记录单和笔, stethoscope if needed 听诊器(按需准备)。

Procedure 操作过程

1. Report and tidy your dress.

报告并整理仪表。

2. Check the validity of hand sanitizer and wash hands in 7 steps and put on the mask.

检查洗手液的有效期，7 步洗手法洗手并戴口罩。

3. Prepare the equipments.

准备用物。

4. Wash hands and remove the mask.

洗手、摘口罩。

5. Take the equipment to the bedside. Evaluate the environment of the ward.

携用物到患者床边。评估病室环境是否适宜操作。

6. Check the patient' s bed number and name. Explain the purpose for the operation.

核对患者床号与姓名。解释操作目的。

7. Assist the patient to appropriate position.

协助患者取合适体位。

8. Select an appropriate site to obtain pulse. The radial pulse is usually taken, place his/her arm in comfortable position.

选择合适的部位测量脉搏。最常用的诊脉部位是桡动脉,将患者手臂置于舒适位置。

9. Palpate the radial artery using the tips of the middle three fingers of your hand with moderate pressure so that you can feel the pulse, note the rhythm and the strength of pulse.

以食指、中指、无名指指端按于桡动脉处,按压力量适中,以能清楚触摸到脉搏的搏动为宜,注意脉搏节律及强弱。

10. If the pulse is regular, count pulse for 30 seconds and multiply by two to obtain pulse rate.

正常脉搏测量 30 s,乘以 2,得出脉率。

11. If the pulse is irregular, count for a full minute. If the pulse is difficult to palpate, auscultate the heart rate for a full minute.

脉率不齐时应测量 1 min。脉搏细弱难触诊时,应听心率 1 min。

12. If a pulse deficit is detected, it should be confirmed by two nurses. One nurse counts the radial pulse while the other nurse auscultates the heart rate. The nurse who is auscultating holds the watch and signals to the other nurse when to start taking pulse and when to stop. Both nurses simultaneously count pulse and heart rate for a full minute.

若发现患者脉搏短绌,应由两名护士同时测量。一人数脉搏,另一人听心率,由听心率者看表并向另一护士发出“起”与“停”的口令,两人同时测量脉搏与心率 1 min。

13. Record the pulse.

记录脉搏情况。

14. Explain the importance of monitoring pulse and tell the related precautions to

the patient.

向患者解释监测脉搏的重要性并告知患者测量脉搏的注意事项。

15. If the pulse is abnormal, observe the related symptoms and signs closely including palpitation and dizzy, and report to your doctor immediately.

如果患者的脉搏异常,应严密观察其伴随症状与体征(包括心悸、头晕等),并及时向医生汇报。

16. Tidy up clothing if necessary.

必要时整理衣服。

17. Tidy up the patient's bed if necessary.

必要时整理床单位。

18. Wash hands.

洗手。

19. Sign the treatment sheet or nursing care plan to indicate that the pulse has been taken.

在治疗单或护理计划单上签名,表示已测量脉搏。

20. Record the pulse rate on the vital sign flowsheet or nursing record according to local policy.

按当地要求在体温单上绘制脉率或在护理记录单上记录。

Nurse Alert 护理事项

1. Note factors that can alter the patient's pulse. Wait 30 minutes before taking pulse if the patient has been acute exercising, stress, fear or crying, etc.

注意有无影响患者脉率变化的因素。若有剧烈运动、紧张、恐惧、哭闹等,应等待30 min后测量。

2. Select an appropriate site for obtaining pulse. Avoid taking pulse on the site with hemiplegia or a wound.

选择合适的脉搏测量部位。避免在偏瘫侧或局部有伤口的部位测量脉搏。

3. Avoid using the thumb for pulse taking because the thumb has pulsation that the nurse could mistake for the patient's pulse.

勿用拇指诊脉,因拇指小动脉搏动易与患者的脉搏相混淆。

4. If the pulse is irregular, count for a full minute. If the pulse is difficult to palpate, double check with heart rate for a full minute. If a pulse deficit is detected, an apical-radial pulse should be taken by two nurses simultaneously for a full minute.

脉率不齐时应测量 1 min。脉搏细弱难触诊时,应复测心率 1 min。若发现患者脉搏短绌,应由 2 名护士同时测量心率和脉率,计时 1 min。

New Words and Expressions
单 词 表

indirectly [ˌindiˈrektli] *adv.* 间接地;不诚实地;迂回地
diagnosis [ˌdaiəgˈnəusis] *n.* 诊断
prevention [priˈvenʃən] *n.* 预防;阻止;妨碍
stethoscope [ˈsteθəˈskəup] *vt.* 用听诊器诊断 *n.* [临床]听诊器
simultaneously [saiməlˈteiniəsli] *adv.* 同时地
precaution [priˈkɔːʃən] *n.* 防范;预防措施;预警

5.3 Assessing Respirations
呼吸的测量

Purpose 操作目的

1. To determine whether the patient's respirations are within normal range.
判断患者的呼吸是否正常。

2. To monitor the changes of respirations dynamically in order to assess the patient's respiratory function.
动态监测呼吸的变化,以了解患者呼吸功能情况。

3. To aid in the diagnosis or to provide data for disease prevention, treatments, rehabilitation and nursing care.
协助诊断或为预防、治疗、康复和护理提供依据。

Assessment 评估

1. Assess the patient's age, level of consciousness, health condition, treatments, medications, psychological status and ability to cooperate.
评估患者的年龄、意识、病情、治疗、用药、心理状态及配合程度。

2. Assess factors that can alter the respiratory rate including acute exercising, excitement or crying, talking respiration-related medications, or received chest surgery or suffered chest trauma.

评估有无影响呼吸频率变化的因素，如是否剧烈运动、情绪激动或哭闹，是否使用影响呼吸的药物，有无胸部手术和外伤史等。

Gather equipment 物品准备

a watch with a second hand 表(有秒针)，record chart and pen 记录单和笔。

Procedure 操作过程

1. Report and tidy your dress.

报告并整理仪表。

2. Check the validity of hand sanitizer and wash hands in 7 steps and put on the mask.

检查洗手液的有效期，7 步洗手法洗手并戴口罩。

3. Prepare the equipments.

准备用物。

4. Wash hands and remove the mask.

洗手、摘口罩。

5. Take the equipment to the bedside. Evaluate the environment of the ward.

携用物到患者床边。评估病室环境是否适宜操作。

6. Check the patient's bed number and name.

核对患者床号与姓名。

7. Assist the patient to appropriate position.

协助患者取合适体位。

8. Distract the patient and encourage the patient to breathe naturally.

转移患者的注意力，使其处于自然呼吸状态。

9. While supposedly taking the radial pulse, observe chest or abdomen rise and fall; or place the patient's arm in relaxed position across the abdomen or chest to feel the patient's chest or abdomen movements.

将手放在患者的桡动脉处于诊脉状，观察患者胸部或腹部的起伏；或让患者手臂放松置于胸部或腹部，感受患者胸部或腹部的起伏运动。

10. Observe the rate, rhythm and depth of respirations, the respiratory sound, the breathing pattern and the effort of breathing. One inhalation/inspiration and one exhalation/expiration count as one respiration.

观察患者呼吸频率、节律、深度、声音、型态及有无呼吸困难等。一吸一呼为一次呼吸。

11. For patients with normal breathing, count respirations for 30 seconds, and multiply by two to obtain pulse rate. For patients with abnormal breathing patterns or for infants, count respirations for a full minute.

正常呼吸患者测量 30 s，乘以 2，得出呼吸频率。异常呼吸患者或婴幼儿应测量 1 min。

12. Record the respirations.

记录呼吸情况。

13. If the patient's respirations are abnormal, observe the related symptoms and signs closely including alteration in consciousness, cyanopathy, count, sputum, emptysis, chest pain, and report to your doctor immediately.

如果患者的呼吸异常，应严密观察伴随症状与体征包括意识改变、发绀、咳嗽、咳痰、咯血、胸痛等，并及时向医生汇报。

14. Tidy up clothing if necessary.

必要时整理衣服。

15. Tidy up the patient's bed if necessary.

必要时整理床单位。

16. Wash hands.

洗手。

17. Sign the treatment sheet or nursing care plan to indicate that the respirations have been taken.

在治疗单或护理计划单上签名，表示已测量呼吸。

18. Record the respiratory rate on the vital sign flowsheet or nursing record according to local policy.

按当地要求在体温单上绘制呼吸频率或在护理记录单上记录。

Nurse Alert 护理事项

1. Note factors that can alter the patient's respirations. Wait 30 minutes before taking respirations if the patient has been acute exercising, excitement or crying, etc.

注意有无影响患者呼吸变化的因素。若有剧烈运动、情绪激动或哭闹等，应等待30 min后测量。

2. Do not let the patient know that you are assessing respirations because this could cause the patient to alter his/her respiratory pattern and you can not obtain accurate respiratory rate.

测量呼吸前不要让患者知道，以免患者改变呼吸型态而不能测得准确的呼吸频率。

3. If the critically ill patient's respirations are too weak to count, place some cotton wool beside his/her nostril, observe the movements of the cotton wool and count respirations for a minute.

如果危重患者呼吸微弱难以测量，可用少许棉絮置于患者鼻孔前，观察棉絮被吹动的次数，并计时1 min。

New Words and Expressions
单 词 表

trauma [ˈtrɔːmə] *n.* 创伤(由心理创伤造成精神上的异常)；外伤
abdomen [ˈæbdəmən] *n.* 腹部
inhalation [ˌinhəˈleiʃən] *n.* 吸入
cyanopathy [ˌsiəˈnɔpəθi] *n.* 发绀
emptysis [ˈemptisis] *n.* 咳血，咯血；吐血

5.4 Assessing Blood Pressure
血压的测量

Purpose 操作目的

1. To determine whether the patient's blood pressure is within normal range.

判断患者的血压是否正常。

2. To monitor the changes of blood pressure dynamically in order to assess the patient's circulatory status indirectly.

动态监测血压变化，间接了解循环系统的功能状况。

3. To aid in the diagnosis or to provide data for disease prevention, treatments,

rehabilitation and nursing care.

协助诊断或为预防、治疗、康复和护理提供依据。

Assessment 评估

1. Assess the patient's age, level of consciousness, health condition, treatments, medications, psychological status and ability to cooperate.

评估患者的年龄、意识、病情、治疗、用药、心理状态及配合程度。

2. Assess factors that can alter the patient's blood pressure, such as smoking, exercising or being exciting.

评估有无影响患者血压的因素，如吸烟、运动、情绪激动等。

3. Assess the patient's mobility and skin condition of limbs and select an appropriate site to obtain blood pressure.

评估患者的肢体功能和皮肤情况，选择适合的测量血压的部位。

Gather equipment 物品准备

tray 治疗盘，sphygmomanometer with appropriate size cuff 袖带规格合适的血压计，stethoscope 听诊器，record chart and pen 记录单和笔。

Procedure 操作过程

1. Report and tidy your dress.

报告并整理仪表。

2. Check the validity of hand sanitizer and wash hands in 7 steps and put on the mask.

检查洗手液的有效期，7 步洗手法洗手并戴口罩。

3. Prepare the equipments. Check the quality of the sphygmomanometer and stethoscope.

准备用物。检查血压计及听诊器的质量。

4. Wash hands and remove the mask.

洗手、摘口罩。

5. Take the equipment to the bedside. Evaluate the environment of the ward.

携用物到患者床边。评估病室环境是否适宜操作。

6. Check the patient's bed number and name. Explain the purpose for the operation.

核对患者床号、姓名。解释操作目的。

7. Assist the patient to appropriate and comfortable position (sitting or lying position) with the forearm (brachial artery) supported at heart level.

协助患者选择合适且舒适的体位(坐位或卧位),使前臂位置(肱动脉)与心脏处于同一水平面上。

8. Expose the patient's upper arm fully, position it with the palm upward and the elbow straight. If the patient's clothing constricts the arm, remove the arm from the sleeve.

充分暴露患者手臂,手掌向上,肘部伸直。如果衣服过紧,则脱下袖子。

9. Open the box of sphygmomanometer and place it on a firm surface and the column of mercury must be placed in an upright position. Open its valve fully, the mercury meniscus is at zero.

打开血压计盒盖,垂直放置平稳。开启水银槽开关,水银柱处于"0"位。

10. Wrap the deflated cuff evenly and snugly around the upper arm so that the center of the bladder is applied directly over the medial aspect of the arm. Place the lower border of the cuff about 2-3 cm above the antecubital fossa/space. Tightness: only one finger can insert into the space under the cuff.

驱净袖带内空气,平整地缠绕于手臂,使袖带气袋中部位于上臂中部。袖带下缘位于肘窝上 2～3 cm,袖带松紧度以能插入 1 指为宜。

11. Instruct the patient not to move or talk during the procedure to avoid false reading.

指导患者测量血压过程中不要移动或讲话,以免影响测量结果。

12. Place the stethoscope earpieces in your ears with it curving slightly forward.

使听诊器耳件稍前倾并戴在耳上。

13. Place the bell/diaphragm of the stethoscope lightly on the medial antecubital fossa where brachial artery pulsations are located with your one hand. With your other hand, close the valve on the pump, and inflate the cuff to a level 20-30 mmHg above the level at which brachial artery pulsations are no longer felt.

一手固定听诊器胸件与肘窝肱动脉搏动最明显处,另一手握加压气球,关闭气门后注气至肱动脉消失再上升 20～30 mmHg。

14. Open the valve on pump, deflate the cuff gradually at the rate of 4 mmHg per second. While observing the sphygmomanometer reading at eye level as the mercury

falls, listen for Korotkoff/thudding sounds of brachial artery pulsations.

打开气门，以 4 mmHg/s 的速度缓慢放气。两眼平视观察水银汞柱缓慢下降，同时听取肱动脉搏动的柯氏音。

15. Note the point on sphygmomanometer when first clear sound is heard which indicates the systolic pressure. Continue to deflate the cuff gradually, note the point on sphygmomanometer at which muffled or dampened sound appears and point at which sound disappears which indicates the diastolic pressure.

留意第一个清晰的搏动音出现时水银柱所指刻度，即为收缩压。继续缓慢放气，留意搏动音突然低钝或消失时水银柱所指刻度，即为舒张压。

16. Open the valve on the pump fully to completely deflate the cuff. Remove it from the patient's arm and tidy up the patient's clothing.

完全打开气门。排尽袖带内余气。取下袖带，整理患者衣服。

17. Place the cuff, pump and tubes in the box of sphygmomanometer. With the sphygmomanometer box 45°, right slantwise to make all mercury go into the trough, close the valve on the box fully and close the sphygmomanometer box.

将袖带、加压气球及胶管置于血压计盒内。右倾血压计 45°，使水银全部流入水银槽，关闭水银槽开关，盖上血压计盒盖。

18. Record the blood pressure reading.

记录血压值。

19. Explain the importance of monitoring blood pressure and inform the patient of related precautions.

向患者解释血压监测的重要性并告知患者测量血压的注意事项。

20. If the blood pressure is abnormal, observe the related symptoms and signs closely including dizziness, headache, flushing, nosebleed, nausea, vomiting, chest tightness, palpitation and limb numbness for hypertension; observe weak and irregular pulse, palpitation and dizziness for hypotension, report to your doctor immediately.

如果患者血压异常，应严密观察其伴随症状和体征包括血压过高时有无头晕、头痛、面色潮红、流鼻血、恶心、呕吐、胸闷、心悸及肢体麻木等，血压过低时有无脉搏细弱或脉率不齐、心悸、头晕等，并及时向医生汇报。

21. Instruct the patient risk factors for high blood pressure, including obesity, increased sodium intake, increased cholesterol intake, smoking and lack of exercise, etc.

告知患者引起高血压的危险因素，包括肥胖、高盐或高胆固醇饮食、吸烟和缺少运动等。

22. For patients taking antihypertensive medications, assess their understanding of the purpose of the medications, explain the importance of maintaining blood pressure and medication adherence.

对于口服降压药的患者，评估他们对用药的目的及重要性的理解情况，并告知他们保持血压平稳及用药依从的重要性。

23. Assist the patient to comfortable position and tidy up clothing.

协助患者取舒适体位，整理衣服。

24. Tidy up the patient's bed if necessary.

必要时整理床单位。

25. Wash hands.

洗手。

26. Sign the treatment sheet or nursing care plan to indicate that the blood pressure has been taken.

在治疗单或护理计划单上签名，表示已测量血压。

27. Record the bloods pressure readings on the vital sign flowsheet or nursing record according to local policy if necessary.

必要时按当地要求在体温单上记录血压值或在护理记录单上记录。

Nurse Alert 护理事项

1. Check the sphygmomanometer periodically to ensure its accuracy. Before assessing a patient's blood pressure, check for chasms or mercury leakages on the glass tube of the sphygmomanometer, check for leakages on its pump and tubes and check the quality of the valve and stethoscope.

定期检测血压计的准确性。测量血压前，需检查血压计的玻璃管有无裂缝，水银有无漏出，加压气球和橡胶管有无漏气，以及气门阀和听诊器的质量是否良好。

2. Note factors that can alter the patient's blood pressure. Wait 30 minutes before blood pressure measurement if the patient has been smoking, exercising, being exciting, etc.

注意有无影响患者血压变化的因素。若有吸烟、运动、情绪激动等，应等待 30 min 后测量。

3. Position the patient's forearm (brachial artery) supported at heart level. If the brachial artery is below the heart level, the blood pressure reading is higher than normal ; and if above the heart level, the reading is lower than normal.

使患者前臂(肱动脉)位置与心脏处于同一水平面上。若肱动脉位置低于心脏,测得的血压值偏高;若其位置高于心脏,测得的血压值偏低。

4. Select a sphygmomanometer with appropriate size cuff according to the patient's age and the site to obtain blood pressure. Cuffs that are too narrow or too wide will cause false high or false low readings respectively. Wrap the deflated cuff evenly and snugly around the upper arm. Cuffs that are wrapped too loose or too tight will cause false high or false low readings respectively.

根据患者的年龄及测量血压的部位,选用袖带规格合适的血压计。袖带过窄或过宽会使测得的血压值偏高或偏低。驱净袖带内空气,平整地缠绕于上臂。袖带缠得过松或过紧也会导致测得的血压值偏高或偏低。

5. If you can not obtain the blood pressure reading or it is out of the normal range, recheck it. Deflate the cuff completely and the mercury meniscus goes to the point of zero, wait a moment before rechecking the blood pressure. Repeat the procedure on his/her other arm if necessary.

发现血压听不清或异常,应重新测量。重测时,应驱尽袖带内的气体,待水银柱降至"0"位,稍等片刻后再测量。必要时做双侧对照。

6. Assess the patient's mobility and the skin of limbs, select an appropriate site to obtain blood pressure.

评估患者的肢体功能和皮肤情况,选择合适的测量血压的部位。

(1) If the patient is receiving intravenous therapy, avoid using the arm that the intravenous cannula or infusion in progress to take blood pressure.

如果患者正接受静脉治疗,应避免在有静脉套管或静脉输液的肢体测量血压。

(2) Avoid measuring blood pressure on an arm with extensive axillary node dissection (e. g. , radical mastectomy) or an arteriovenous fistula (e. g. , for dialysis).

避免在进行腋窝淋巴结清扫(乳癌根治术时)或有动静脉瘘(透析时)的肢体上测量血压。

(3) Avoid measuring blood pressure on an extremity with trauma, paralysis or paresis.

避免在有外伤、偏瘫或麻痹的肢体上测量血压。

7. For patients who need close blood pressure monitoring, take blood pressure at specified time, on the same site, with the same position and by the same sphygmomanometer for accuracy and contrast.

对需要密切观察血压的患者,应定时间、定部位、定体位、定血压计测量,这样有助于测量的准确性和对照的可比性。

New Words and Expressions
单 词 表

forearm [fɔːrɑːm] *n.* 前臂
antecubital fossa *n.* 肘窝
dizziness [ˈdizinis] *n.* 头晕
hypertension [ˈhaipəuˈtenʃən] *n.* 高血压

Communication Model
沟 通 模 板

Self-introduction Model 常规介绍模板

Good morning/afternoon teachers, my name is ××, I come from class ××, my student's number is ××. Today, I am going to show you the process of measuring vital signs, the equipments I have prepared are. . . ,everything is ready, may I start?

老师上午好/下午好。我是××,来自××班,我的学号是××。今天我要展示的操作是生命体征测量,准备的用物有……,准备完毕,请求开始。

Assessment 评估

The environment is tidy and comfortable. It's suitable for the procedure.

环境整洁舒适,适宜操作。

Communication 沟通

Hello, I'm your primary nurse, my name is ××. Would you tell me your full name? How do you feel now? How long have you been in bed? Well, I will assess the vital signs for you. It includes temperature, pulse blood and blood pressure. Since you are newly admitted, have you ever measure these?

您好,我是您的责任护士,我的名字是××。可以告诉我您的名字吗?您现在感觉怎么样？您卧床多长时间了？我将为您测量生命体征，包括体温、脉搏和血压。因您是新入院的，以前测量过吗？

1. Temperature 体温

(1) Oral temperature: Did you drink any hot water or eat hot food in the last half an hour? OK, good, please put the thermometer under your tongue.

口温：请问您半小时内喝过热饮或吃过热的食物吗？好的，请将口表水银端放于舌下热窝处。

(2) Axillary temperature: Do you have sweat in your armpit? I will clean it for you. Please put the thermometer under your armpit.

腋温：请问您腋下有汗吗？我将为您擦拭。请将体温计水银端放在腋窝中央，并屈臂过胸夹紧。

(3) Rectal temperature: Please take off your trousers to the knee and tune left, keep this position for 3 minutes. You will feel a little pain when I insert the thermometer into your anus, please don't move!

肛温：请您脱下裤子至膝盖处并向左侧卧，保持这个体位 3 min。当我将肛表插入您的肛门时您可能会感觉到一点点不适，请不要动。

2. Pulse 脉搏

Please give me your hand, I will check your pulse rate.

请伸出您的手，我将为您测量脉率。

(Patient: How is my pulse rate?)

(患者：我的脉率是多少?)

A little bit fast, but the rhythm is normal. That means your heart is pumping regularly without skipping. / It is in the normal range.

有一点快，但节律正常。这表示您的心脏搏动规律无漏跳/在正常范围内。

3. Blood Pressure 血压

Please roll up your sleeve and get to the elbow. Do you feel tight? OK, your blood pressure is in the normal range.

请您将袖子挽至肘部以上。您感觉紧吗？好，您的血压在正常范围内。

OK, your temperature is ××, your pulse is ××, your BP is××. They all indicate that your body is in good condition, and I am sure you will recover soon. Have a good rest. See you!

您的体温是××，您的脉率是××，您的血压是××。这些数据提示您的身体状态不错，我相信您会很快康复。好好休息，再见！

Scoring Criteria 7
评分细则 7

项目		总分	技术操作要求	标准分	扣分说明	得分
评估 12	仪表	4	仪表端庄、服装整洁、修剪指甲、洗手、戴口罩	4	一项不符扣 2 分	
	物品	4	用物齐备,放置合理,全面检查用物完好性	2	一项不符扣 2 分	
	环境		环境符合要求	2		
	患者	4	根据情况全面评估(情绪、运动、饮食、冷热、出汗、配合情况、病情、基础血压等)	4	一项不符扣 1 分	
实施 68	核对解释	4	核对床号、姓名	2	一项不符扣 2 分	
			解释内容合理(操作目的、配合方法及注意事项)	2	一项不符扣 2 分	
	体温测量	8	擦去腋窝汗液,夹体温计(摆放上臂姿势)方法正确	4	一项不符扣 2 分	
			测量时间充分,读数准确	4	一项不符扣 2 分	
	脉搏测量	10	示指、中指、无名指指端按压桡动脉处,以清除触到脉搏搏动为宜,计数 30 s,计数乘以 2	6	一项不符扣 2 分	
			测量时间充分,计数准确	4	一项不符扣 2 分	
	呼吸测量	8	脉搏测量结束后,手仍保持诊断状态,眼睛观察胸部或腹部起伏	4	一项不符扣 2 分	
			计数 30 s,计数乘以 2	4	一项不符扣 2 分	
	血压测量	30	合适体位,卷袖,手掌向上,肘部伸直	4	一项不符扣 2 分	
			被测肢体放置(高度、角度)合理	2	一项不符扣 2 分	
			血压计放置合理(高度、竖直)	2	一项不符扣 2 分	
			打开血压计垂直,放妥,并打开水银槽开关	2	一项不符扣 1 分	
			缠袖带(在肘窝上 2~3 cm),试松紧(1 指为宜)	4	一项不符扣 2 分	
			触摸肱动脉,将听诊器加温并置于肱动脉最明显处	2	一项不符扣 2 分	
			注气至肱动脉的搏动消失后再上升 20~30 mmHg,缓慢放气(4 mmHg/s)	4	差 2 mmHg/s 扣 3 分,超过扣 4 分	
			正确读数,眼睛视线保持与水银柱弯月面同一水平	4	一项不符扣 2 分	
			整理血压计:驱尽袖带内的空气,血压计盒右倾 45°,水银全部流入水银槽内,关闭水银开关,盖上盒盖,平稳放置	4	差 8 mmHg/s 扣 1 分,超过扣 4 分	
			测量结果正确(误差<4 mmHg)	2	一项不符扣 2 分	
	整理	8	患者体位舒适,衣物整洁	2	一项不符扣 2 分	
			床单位整洁	2	一项不符扣 2 分	
			用物处理正确(浸泡、毁形),洗手并记录	4	一项不符扣 2 分	

续表

项目		总分	技术操作要求	标准分	扣分说明	得分
评价 20	熟练	8	动作轻稳、熟练，步骤合理	2	一项不符扣 2 分	
			相关理论知识掌握熟练	2	一项不符扣 2 分	
			按规定时间完成(10 min)，职业保护恰当	4	一项不符扣 2 分	
	效果	2	患者感觉安全舒适，无不良反应	2	酌情扣分	
	英语	10	发音准确，语言流畅，关爱患者，沟通良好	10	酌情扣分	
主考教师：		日期：		总分：100	得分：	

评分标准：91～100 分为优，81～90 分为良，71～80 分为中，60～70 分为差，低于 60 分为不及格。

Chapter 6 Administering Oxygen and Suctioning 吸氧吸痰法

6.1 Administering Oxygen by a Nasal Catheter 鼻导管给氧法

Purpose 操作目的

1. To increase arterial partial pressure of oxygen (PaO_2) and arterial oxyhemoglobin saturation(SaO_2) in patients with hypoxemia.

用于各种缺氧的患者以提高动脉血氧分压(PaO_2)和动脉血氧饱和度(SaO_2)。

2. To promote patient's metabolism and maintain life's activities.

促进组织的新陈代谢,维持机体的生命活动。

Assessment 评估

1. Assess the patient's age, level of consciousness, health condition, the causes and degree of hypoxemia.

评估患者的年龄、意识、病情、缺氧原因及程度。

2. Assess the condition of the patient's nasal cavity including deviation of nasal septum or damaged mucosa, etc.

评估患者鼻腔的情况,包括有无鼻中隔弯曲或黏膜损伤等。

3. Assess the patient's experience and understanding of oxygen therapy and its plan.

评估患者的氧疗经历及对氧疗知识、氧疗计划的了解程度。

4. Assess the patient's psychological status, ability to cooperate and communication skills.

评估患者的心理状态、配合程度及表达能力。

Gather equipment 物品准备

1. 治疗车上层

治疗盘内:sterile bowl with cold boiled water 治疗碗(内盛冷开水),gauzes 纱布,nasal catheter 鼻导管,sterile swabs 棉签,adhesive tape 胶布。

治疗盘外:prescription chart 医嘱单,kidney basin 弯盘,oxygen equipment 氧气装置(pressure gauge 压力表、flowmeter 流量表、humidifier bottle with sterile water 湿化瓶(内盛无菌水),record chart 记录单,pen 笔,hand sanitizer 洗手液。

2. 治疗车下层

medical waste bin 医用垃圾桶,household garbage bin 生活垃圾桶。

Procedure 操作过程

1. Report and tidy your dress.

报告并整理仪表。

2. Check the validity of hand sanitizer and wash hands in 7 steps and put on the mask.

检查洗手液的有效期,7 步洗手法洗手并戴口罩。

3. Gather and check equipments.

备齐并检查用物。

4. Wash hands and remove the mask.

洗手、摘口罩。

5. Assess the environment. No pyrotechnical, tinder and smoking in the ward.

评估环境。病室无火源和易燃物品,无人吸烟。

6. Take the equipment to the bedside. Check the patient's bed number and name. Explain the purpose of the operation.

携用物至患者床旁。核对患者床号与姓名。解释操作目的。

7. Check the patient's nasal cavity including deviation of nasal septum or damaged mucosa, etc.

检查患者鼻腔的情况,包括有无鼻中隔弯曲或黏膜损伤等。

8. Assist the patient to semi-Fowler's position if possible.

摆体位,如有可能,协助患者取半坐卧位。

9. Wash hand and put on a mask.

洗手、戴口罩。

10. Clean the patient's nasal cavities with swabs.

用棉签清洁鼻孔。

11. Attach the flowmeter to the wall outlet, exerting firm pressure. Turn on the flowmeter, check whether the tubing is patent and whether the connections are airtight, and then close it.

用力将流量表安装到墙上的氧气气源插座上。打开流量开关,检查氧气流通是否通畅,有无漏气,然后关闭流量开关。

12. Connect a nasal catheter with the export of humidifier.

将鼻导管与湿化瓶的出口相连接。

13. Turn on the flowmeter at the flow rate ordered.

打开流量开关,根据医嘱调节氧流量。

14. Insert the tip of the nasal catheter into a sterile blow with cold boiled water to moisten the tip and to test the oxygen flow.

将鼻导管的前端置于无菌治疗碗的凉开水中,湿润管前端并检查氧气流出情况。

15. Place the nasal catheter in the patient's nostrils. Position the tubing over and behind each ear, and slide the adjuster under the chin so that the nasal catheter fits snugly and comfortably.

将鼻导管插入患者鼻孔。将导管两端环绕患者耳后向下,在下巴下调节导管松紧度,使之固定得松紧适宜且舒适。

16. Providing health education

(1) Warn the patient and visitors not to adjust the flow rate of oxygen spontaneously.

提醒患者及探访者不要自行调节氧流量。

(2) Warn the patient any visitors to follow the "four safety precautions" when using oxygen.

提醒患者及探访者遵守氧疗"四防"。

(3) Instruct the patient to keep the tubing patent.

指导患者保持管道通畅。

(4) Ask the patient to notify nurse immediately whenever any unusual effects are occurring.

告知患者若有不适立即告知护士。

(5) Instruct the patient how to use call signal and have it within patient's reach.

指导患者使用呼叫器,并将呼叫器放于易取处。

17. Assist the patient to comfortable position.

协助患者取舒适体位。

18. Record the initiation time of oxygen therapy, flow rate and the patient's response to oxygen.

记录氧疗开始时间、氧流量及患者的反应。

19. Assess the patient periodically for clinical signs of hypoxia: confusion, cyanosis, dyspnea, tachycardia, and restlessness, etc.

定时评估患者有无缺氧情况,如意识模糊、脸色苍白、呼吸困难、心动过速及烦躁不安等。

20. Discontinuing oxygen therapy.

停止氧疗。

(1) Remove the nasal catheter, discard the nasal catheter into the kidney basin or medical waste receiver.

拔出鼻导管,将鼻导管放于弯盘或医用垃圾袋内。

(2) Unload the regulator from the wall outlet if necessary.

必要时卸表。

(3) Perform nasal hygiene.

拭净患者鼻部。

21. Assist the patient to comfortable position.

协助患者取舒适体位。

22. Wash hand and sign the prescription chart or treatment sheet to indicate that the oxygen therapy has been discontinued.

洗手并在医嘱单或治疗单上签名,表示已停止氧疗。

23. Document the effectiveness of the oxygen therapy and discontinued time.

记录氧疗效果及停氧时间。

Nurse Alert 护理事项

1. Observe the procedure of oxygen therapy, especially paying attention to the "four safety precautions for oxygen administration" to prevent fire.

应遵守氧疗操作规程,尤其是注意做好"四防用氧安全措施"以预防火灾。

2. Ensure that oxygen is flowing freely through the tubing. There should be no kinks in the tubing, and the connections should be airtight to avoid leakage of oxygen.

确保管道通畅,没有扭曲,接口密封良好,无氧气泄露。

3. When initiating oxygen therapy, regulate the flow rate before oxygen is supplied. When terminating oxygen therapy, remove the catheter or cannula before turning off the flowmeter. If you need to change the flow rate for your patient, separate the catheter or cannula from the humidifier bottle, adjust to a new flow rate and then connect them.

使用氧气时,应先调节流量后使用。停用氧气时,应先拔除鼻导管再关流量开关。中途调节流量时,应先分离鼻导管与湿化瓶连接处,调节好流量再接上。

4. Regulate the flow rate of oxygen according to doctor's order or the patient's condition.

根据医嘱或患者病情调节氧流量。

5. Sterile water is commonly used to humidify oxygen. 20%-30% alcohol may be used for patients with acute pulmonary edema.

常用无菌液为无菌水。急性肺水肿时用20%～30%酒精。

6. Moniter the patient closely while he/she is on oxygen therapy. Disconnect the oxygen temporarily to prevent aspiration when the patient is drinking or eating.

氧疗过程中应加强监测。患者饮水或进食时,应暂停吸氧以防误吸。

New Words and Expressions
单 词 表

administer [əd'ministə] *vt.* 管理;执行;给予

oxygen ['ɔksidʒən] *n.* [化学] 氧气,[化学]氧

nasal ['neizəl] *adj.* 鼻的

catheter ['kæθitə] *n.* [医] 导管;导尿管;尿液管

arterial [ɑː'tiəriəl] *adj.* [解剖] 动脉的;干线的;似动脉的

partial [ˈpɑːʃəl] *adj*. 局部的

oxyhemoglobin [ˌɔksiˌhiːməuˈgləubin] *n*. 氧基血红素；氧合血红蛋白

saturation [sætʃəˈreiʃən] *n*. 饱和；色饱和度；浸透；磁化饱和

hypoxemia [ˌhaipɔkˈsiːmiə] *n*. 血氧不足，低氧血症

metabolism [meˈtæbəlizəm] *n*. [生理] 新陈代谢

cavity [ˈkæviti] *n*. 腔；洞，凹处

deviation [ˈdiːviˈeiʃən] *n*. 偏差；误差；背离

septum [ˈseptəm] *n*. 隔膜

mucosa [mjuːˈkəusə] *n*. [解剖]黏膜

adhesive [ədˈhiːsiv] *adj*. 黏着的；带黏性的

humidifier [hjuːˈmidiˌfaiə] *n*. 增湿器，[建] 加湿器

pyrotechnical [ˌpairəuˈteknikl] *n*. 烟火装置 adj. 烟火的

tinder [ˈtində] *n*. 火绒；易燃物

nostril [ˈnɔstril] *n*. 鼻孔

snugly [ˈsnʌgli] *adv*. 舒适地；贴身地；紧密地

spontaneously [spɔnˈteiniəsli] *adv*. 自发地；自然地；不由自主地

precaution [priˈkɔːʃən] *n*. 防范；预防措施；预警

periodically [piəriˈɔdikəli] *adv*. 定期地；周期性地；偶尔

confusion [kənˈfjuːʒən] *n*. 混淆，混乱；困惑

cyanosis [ˌsaiəˈnəusis] *n*. 苍白病；黄萎病

dyspnea [ˈdispniə] *n*. [内科] 呼吸困难

tachycardia [ˌtækiˈkaːdiə] *n*. [内科] 心动过速；心跳过速

restlessness [ˈrestəisnəs] *n*. 坐立不安；不安定

hygiene [ˈhaidʒiːn] *n*. 卫生；卫生学；保健法

Communication Model
沟 通 模 板

Self-introduction Model 常规介绍模板

Good morning/afternoon teachers, my name is ××, I come from class ××, my student's number is ××. Today, I am going to show you the process of administering oxygen, the equipments I have prepared are ... ,everything is ready, may I start?

老师上午/下午好，我是××，来自××班，我的学号是××。今天我要展示的操作是吸氧术，所准备的用物有……，准备完毕，请求开始。

Assessment 评估

The ward is tidy and well ventilated. The patient is in good mental state, he has ability to cooperate with me.

病室整洁、通风良好。患者精神状态良好，有配合操作的能力。

Communication 沟通

Nurse: Good morning /afternoon sir. May I have your name? OK, Mr ××, I'm××, I'm your duty nurse today. How are you feeling now?

护士：早上/下午好，先生，请问你叫什么名字？好的，××先生，我是你的责任护士，我叫××，您现在感觉怎么样？

Patient: I feel a little shortness of breath.

患者：我现在感觉有点气短。

Nurse: According to the doctor's order, I will administering oxygen for you. It can relieve your breathing difficulty and shortness of breath. Don't worry. When you feel better we will remove the catheter. So, would you like to cooperate with me?

护士：遵医嘱，我要给您氧气吸入。这能够减轻您的呼吸困难和气短的症状。别担心，如果您感觉好点了，我会为您移除鼻导管的。您能配合我的操作吗？

Patient: OK.

患者：当然。

Nurse: Thank you.

护士：谢谢。

Assessment 评估

Nurse: I will check your nose, don't be nervous. It doesn't be hurt. There is no deviation of nasal septum. The nasal mucosa is in good condition. Have you ever done the nasal operation before?

护士：我要为您检查鼻腔，别紧张，不疼。没有鼻中隔的偏移，鼻黏膜状态良好。您以前做过鼻腔手术吗？

Patient：No.

患者：没有。

Nurse：Are you having a stuffy nose or some other discomforts now?

护士：您现在有没有鼻腔不通气或其他的不适？

Patient：No，I am fine.

患者：没有，我感觉很好。

Positioning　取体位

Nurse：Would you prefer to lay in bed or to sit up?

护士：您想躺着还是坐起来？

Patient：I think lay in bed is good.

患者：我想还是躺着好点。

Nurse：OK，I will help you. Do you feel comfortable?

护士：好的，我来帮您。您感觉舒服吗？

Patient：Yes，of course.

患者：是的。

Cleaning　清洁

Nurse：I will clean your nose. You will feel a little cold.

护士：我要为您清洁鼻腔，您会感觉有点凉。

Health education　健康教育

Nurse：How do you feel now? I've done the procedure. Now，listen to me carefully. Please don't adjust the oxygen flow by yourself and keep the tubing patent. And no fire，no smoking near the oxygen. Are you clear about that? OK，very well. If you need any help，please press the button on the call signal. I will be here as soon as possible. Have a good rest. See you then.

护士：您现在感觉怎么样？我已经为您上好鼻导管了。现在请认真听我讲。您自己不要随意调节氧流量，请保持导管的通畅。用氧时请勿在附近用明火或者吸烟。您都明确了吗？好的，很好。如果您有其他的需要，请按呼叫器，我会尽快来看您的。好好休息，再见。

Remove the nasal catheter　移除鼻导管

Nurse：How are you feeling now?

护士：您现在感觉怎么样？

Patient：I feel very well.

患者：我感觉非常好。

Nurse：According to the doctor's order，I will remove the catheter for you. Let me help you. Do you feel comfortable in this position? If you need any help. Let me know. Please press the button on the call signal. I will be here as soon as possible. I'd love to help you. See you!

护士:根据医嘱,我现在要为您停止吸氧。我来帮您。您现在感觉这个体位舒适吗?如果您有其他的需要,请按呼叫器通知我,我会尽快来看您的,很高兴能帮助您,再见!

Scoring Criteria 8
评分细则 8

项目		总分	技术操作要求	标准分	扣分说明	得分
评估 10	仪表	2	仪表端庄、服装整洁、修剪指甲、洗手、戴口罩	2	一项不符扣 1 分	
	物品	6	用物齐备，治疗车上、下放置合理	4	一项不符扣 1 分	
	环境		环境符合要求	2	一项不符扣 2 分	
	患者	2	了解患者病情、缺氧程度、配合程度	2	一项不符扣 1 分	
实施 70	核对解释	6	核对床号、姓名	2	一项不符扣 2 分	
			解释操作目的及配合方法，评估患者鼻腔情况	4	一项不符扣 2 分	
	准备氧气	4	正确安装流量表	2	一项不符扣 2 分	
			开流量表，检查氧气表是否通畅，关流量表	2	一项不符扣 2 分	
	吸氧	30	协助患者取舒适体位	2	一项不符扣 2 分	
			选择并清洁鼻腔(单鼻腔或双鼻腔)	2	一项不符扣 1 分	
			检查并连接鼻导管正确	4	一项不符扣 2 分	
			根据病情需要正确调节氧气流量	4	一项不符扣 2 分	
			鼻导管试通畅、湿润	4	一项不符扣 2 分	
			插鼻导管方法正确，深度合适	2	一项不符扣 2 分	
			导管固定适宜	2	一项不符扣 2 分	
			协助患者取舒适体位	2	一项不符扣 2 分	
			健康教育合理(不可自行调节氧流量，要确保鼻导管通畅，做好“四防”，如有不适及时沟通。)	6	一项不符扣 2 分	
			记录用氧时间、患者反应等	2	一项不符扣 1 分	
	停止吸氧	20	评估缺氧改善情况，向患者解释停止吸氧原因	4	一项不符扣 2 分	
			解除固定	2	一项不符扣 2 分	
			取纱布于手中，摘下鼻塞，清洁患者面部	4	一项不符扣 2 分	
			关流量表，弃鼻导管于污物桶中	2	一项不符扣 2 分	
			卸表方法正确，放置于车下层	2	一项不符扣 2 分	
			安置患者于舒适体位	2	一项不符扣 2 分	
			记录停氧时间、患者的反应	4	一项不符扣 2 分	
	操作后整理	10	患者卧位舒适，衣物整洁，床单位整洁	2	一项不符扣 1 分	
			用物处理正确	4	一项不符扣 2 分	
			洗手、记录	4	一项不符扣 2 分	
评价 20	熟练	8	动作轻柔、熟练、步骤合理	2	一项不符扣 2 分	
			检查各种物品有效期，遵守无菌原则	2	一项不符扣 2 分	
			相关理论知识掌握熟练	2	酌情扣分	
			按规定时间完成(5 min)	2	每超过 30 s 扣 1 分	
	效果	2	患者感觉安全舒适	2	酌情扣分	
	沟通	10	英语发音准确，语言流畅，关爱患者，沟通良好	10	酌情扣分	

主考教师：	日期：	总分：100	得分：

评分标准：91～100 分为优，81～90 分为良，71～80 分为中，60～70 分为差，低于 60 分为不及格。

6.2 Suctioning
吸 痰 法

Purpose 操作目的

1. To remove secretions from the respiratory tract in order to maintain a patient airway.

清除呼吸道分泌物,保持呼吸道通畅。

2. To promote gas exchange in order to relieve breathing difficulty.

改善气体交换,缓解呼吸困难。

Assessment 评估

1. Assess the patient's age, level of consciousness, health condition and his/her treatments, especially assess whether the patient is unable to cough or swallow, or he/she presents the signs and symptoms of secretions accumulation or hypoxia.

评估患者的年龄、意识、病情及治疗情况,尤其注意评估患者有无咳嗽及吞咽能力、有无痰液聚集及缺氧的症状、体征。

2. Assess the condition of the patient's oral and nasal cavity whether there are moveable dentures or deviation of nasal septum.

评估患者口腔及鼻腔的情况,有无活动义齿或鼻中隔弯曲。

3. Assess the patient's psychological status, ability to cooperate and communication skills.

评估患者的心理状态、合作程度及表达能力。

Gather equipment 物品准备

1. 治疗车上层

治疗盘内:sterile disposable suction catheters 一次性无菌吸痰管,sterile gauzes 消毒纱布,sterile swabs 无菌棉签,sterile forceps 无菌镊子,drape 治疗巾,PE gloves PE 手套,iodophor 碘伏,sterile container with normal saline 无菌缸(内盛生理盐水),adhesive tape 胶布,tongue blade, mouth gag and tongue forceps if necessary 压舌板、

张口器、舌钳(按需准备)。

治疗盘外：prescription chart 医嘱单、portable electrical suction machine or wall-mounted suction unit 电动吸引器或中心吸引器、pressure gauge 压力表、suctionbottle 储液瓶，kidney basin 弯盘，hand sanitizer 洗手液。

2. 治疗车下层

medical waste bin 医用垃圾桶，household garbage bin 生活垃圾桶。

Procedure 操作过程

1. Report and tidy your dress.

报告并整理仪表。

2. Check the validity of hand sanitizer and wash hands in 7 steps and put on the mask.

检查洗手液的有效期，7 步洗手法洗手并戴口罩。

3. Gather and check equipments.

备齐并检查用物。

4. Wash hands and remove the mask.

洗手、摘口罩。

5. Assess the working environment is clean and quiet with adequate lighting and space.

评估操作环境清洁、安静，光线充足，空间宽敞。

6. Take the equipment to the bedside. Check the patient's bed number and name. Explain the purpose of suctioning and get cooperation.

携用物到患者床边。核对患者床号和姓名。解释吸痰目的并取得患者合作。

7. Wash hands and put on a mask.

洗手、戴口罩。

8. Assess the condition of the patient's oral and nasal cavity. For the unconscious patient, open his/her mouth with a tongue blade or a mouth gag. Remove the moveable dentures. Doing lung auscultation on the same place of both side of the chest walls if necessary.

评估患者口腔及鼻腔情况，昏迷患者可用压舌板或开口器协助开口，取下活动义齿。必要时双侧胸壁上方进行肺部听诊。

9. Assist the patient to lay on back with the patient's head turned to one side and facing you.

协助患者取仰卧位，头偏向一侧，面向操作者。

10. Place a kidney basin near the corner of the mouth.

置弯盘于患者口角旁。

11. Plug in and switch on the electrical suction machine, check its function. Set desired pressure. In general, 40.0-53.3 kPa is used for adults, 33.0-40.0 kPa for children.

接通电源，打开电动吸引器开关，检查其性能，调节负压。一般成人 40.0～53.3 kPa，儿童 33.0～40.0 kPa。

12. Open the cover of the sterile container.

打开无菌缸盖。

13. Check and open the sterile suction catheter package, take out the drape and place the drape under the patient's chin to protect his/her gown and pillow.

检查并打开无菌吸痰管包装，取出治疗巾，颌下铺治疗巾以保护患者衣服及枕头。

14. Wear gloves in right hand.

戴手套于右手。

15. Attach the catheter to the tubing of suction machine.

将吸痰管连接到吸引器的连接管上。

16. Moisten the catheter tip by dipping it in sterile NS.

将吸痰管前端浸入无菌生理盐水，以达到润湿的目的。

17. Test the suction and the patency of the catheter by sucking a small amount of sterile NS.

试吸少量生理盐水，以检查有无吸力及吸痰管是否通畅。

18. Insert the suction catheter for suctioning.

插入吸痰管进行吸痰。

(1) For an oropharyngeal suction, insert the catheter through the mouth into oropharynx (10-15cm) without applying suction.

口咽部吸痰：不带负压将吸痰管从口腔插入口咽部(10～15 cm)。

(2) For a nasopharyngeal suction, insert the catheter gently through one nostril without applying suction. If one nostril is not patent, try the other one.

鼻咽部吸痰：不带负压将吸痰管轻轻从一侧鼻腔插入。如果一侧鼻腔不通畅，则插另一侧。

(3) Begin suctioning by using a rotating motion as the catheter is being withdrawn. Apply intermittent suction for up to 15 seconds.

开始吸痰，采取左右旋转并向上提管的手法。每次吸痰时间不超过 15 s。

19. Flushing the catheter when the catheter has been removed, flush the catheter with sterile NS.

吸痰管退出后,用无菌生理盐水冲管。

20. If necessary, repeat the procedure using a new catheter until the airway is clear.

必要时更换吸痰管重复抽吸,直至气道痰液被吸干净为止。

21. Turn off the suction machine. Discard the used catheter into the medical waste bag.

关吸引器。将用过的吸痰管放入医用垃圾袋内。

22. Cover the head of the tube with gauzes.

用纱布将连接管头端包好。

23. Observe the patient's response to suctioning. Assess lung sounds, heart rate and rhythm for changes. Observe the amount, consistency, color and odor of secretions.

观察患者对吸痰的反应,评估呼吸音、心率、心律的变化。观察吸出痰液的量、黏稠度、颜色、气味。

24. Perform oral or nasal hygiene if necessary.

必要时拭净患者口鼻。

25. Assist the patient to comfortable position and tidy up clothing if necessary.

协助患者取舒适卧位,必要时整理衣服。

26. Ask the patient's feelings and needs.

询问患者的感受及需求。

27. Encourage the patient to cough and expectorate secretions if possible. Ask the patient to notify nurse immediately whenever any unusual effects are occurring. Instruct the patient how to use call signal and have it within patient's reach.

如有可能,鼓励患者咳嗽、排痰。告诉患者若有不适立即告知护士。指导患者正确使用呼叫器,并置于易取处。

28. Discard all used equipment appropriately.

合理清理用物。

29. Wash hands and remove the mask.

洗手、摘口罩。

30. Observing and recording 观察并记录

(1) Continue to observe the patient's breathing status closely.

继续严密观察患者的呼吸情况。

(2) Evaluate the desired effect of suctioning. Record the route used to suction, frequency of suctioning, secretions obtained, amount, consistency, color and odor of secretions, and the patient's response, etc.

评价吸痰效果。记录吸痰途径、吸痰的频率、抽吸出的分泌物及其量、黏稠度、颜色、气味和患者的反应等。

Nurse Alert 护理事项

1. Before suctioning, check the condition of electrical suction machine or wall-mounted suction unit and attach the suction tubing correctly.

吸痰前,检查电动吸引器或中心吸引器的性能并正确连接管道。

2. Observe aseptic technique strictly. For tracheotomy patients, insert the suction catheter into the tracheotomy tube first, and then oropharynx and nasopharynx. One sterile catheter is required for each time.

严格遵守无菌技术操作原则。对气管切开患者,应先吸气管切开处,再吸口咽部、鼻咽部,且每吸痰一次应更换吸痰管。

3. In order to prevent trauma to the respiratory mucosa, insert the catheter without applying suction, and use gentle action while suctioning.

为了防止呼吸道黏膜损伤,插管时不能带负压,吸痰动作应轻柔。

4. Prevent hypoxia due to prolonged suction. Apply intermittent suction for up to 15 seconds.

避免抽吸时间过长造成缺氧。每次吸痰时间不超过 15 s。

5. For patients with mucous plugs, perform inhalation and percussion on the back to improve the effect of suctioning.

痰液黏稠时,应给予雾化吸入,可配合背部叩击,以提高吸痰的效果。

6. Empty the suction bottle before the content inside reaches to two-thirds full.

储液瓶内吸出液不得超过 2/3,应及时倾倒。

New Words and Expressions
单 词 表

suction [ˈsʌkʃən] *n.* 吸;吸力;抽吸

secretion [siˈkriːʃən] *n.* 分泌;分泌物;藏匿;隐藏

respiratory [riˈspaiərtəri] *adj.* 呼吸的

swallow [ˈswɔləu] *vi.* 吞下；咽下
symptom [ˈsim(p)təm] *n.* [临床] 症状；征兆
accumulation [əˌkjuːmjuˈleiʃən] *n.* 积聚，累积；堆积物
hypoxia [haiˈpɔksiə] *n.* [医] 低氧；组织缺氧；氧不足
portable [ˈpɔːtəbl] *adj.* 手提的，便携式的；轻便的
auscultation [ˌɔːskəlˈteiʃən] *n.* 听；[医学] 听诊(法)
plug [plʌg] *vi.* 塞住
desired [diˈzaiəd] *adj.* 渴望的；想得到的
oropharyngeal [ˈɔːrəufærinˈdʒiːəl] *adj.* 口咽的
oropharynx [ˌɔːrəuˈfæriŋks] *n.* [解剖]口咽
nasopharyngeal [neizəuˌfærinˈdʒiːəl] *adj.* 鼻咽的
rotate [rəuˈteit] *vi.* 旋转；循环
withdrawn [wiðˈdrɔːn] *v.* 取出；撤退(withdraw 的过去分词)
intermittent [ˌintəˈmitənt] *adj.* 间歇的，断断续续的
consistency [kənˈsistənsi] *n.* 稠度；稠厚度
expectorate [eksˈpektəreit] *vt.* 咳出痰；吐唾液；咯血

Communication Model
沟通模板

Self-introduction Model 常规介绍模板

Good morning/afternoon teachers, my name is ××, I come from class ××, my student's number is ××. Today, I am going to show you the process of suctioning, the equipments I have prepared are ..., everything is ready, may I start?

老师上午/下午好，我是××，来自××班，我的学号是××。今天我要展示的操作是吸痰术，所准备的用物有……，准备完毕，请求开始。

Assessment 评估

The ward is tidy and well ventilated. The patient is unconscious, he is unable to cough or swallow, or he presents the signs and symptoms of secretions accumulation and hypoxia.

病室整洁、通风良好，患者意识模糊，没有咳嗽及吞咽能力，有痰液聚集及缺氧的症状和体征。

Communication 沟 通

Good morning, sir. I'm your duty nurse. If you speak difficulty, you can nod or shake your head. Are you ××(the patient's name)? OK, Mr ××. Do you have secretions in your throat and feel dyspnea?

早上好，先生，我是您今天的责任护士，如果您说话困难，亲点头或摇手示意我。请问您是××吗？好的，××先生，您咽喉部有很多分泌物并感觉呼吸困难吗？

Please open your mouth (open up). Let me check it.

请张开嘴，让我来检查一下。

OK, there are no dentures, deviation of nasal septum. OK, very well. Let me help you to auscultate your lung. There are a lot of secretion accumulate in your respiratory tract. So I will help you to remove it in order to maintain your airway. Would you please cooperate with me. If you have unbearable discomfort, please let me know, and I'll do it gently.

好的，没有义齿，没有鼻中隔偏移。好的，非常好。让我来帮您做肺部的听诊。有大量的痰液聚集在呼吸道。所以我要帮您清除分泌物来保证呼吸道通畅，请配合我的操作。如果在过程中有难以忍受的不适，请示意我，我会动作轻柔些的。

Positioning 取体位

I'll turn you to the supine position with your head facing me.

我要为您取仰卧位头偏一侧。

Suctioning 吸痰

I will insert the suction catheter for suctioning, You may feel discomfort, just like cough. Take it easy, relax.

我要插入吸痰管来吸痰了，您会感觉有些不适，例如咳嗽，请您放松，别紧张。

Observing 观察

Observe the patient's response. Assess lung sounds, heart rate and rhythm for changes. Observe the amount, consistency, color and odor of secretions.

观察患者的反应，评估患者的呼吸音、心率及节律有无变化。观察痰液的量、黏稠度、颜色及气味。

Health education 健康教育

Do you feel comfortable now? OK, do you feel comfortable in this position? It's

good for you to drink water regularly. OK, if you need any help, please press the button on the call signal. I'll come here as soon as possible. Have a good rest. See you!

您现在感觉舒适吗？好的，这个体位您觉得舒适吗？经常喝水对您是有好处的。如果您有任何的不适，请按呼叫器呼叫我，我会尽快来看您的，好好休息，再见！

Scoring Criteria 9
评分细则 9

项目		总分	技术操作要求	标准分	扣分说明	得分
评估 10	仪表	2	仪表端庄、服装整洁、修剪指甲、洗手、戴口罩	2	一项不符扣 1 分	
	物品	6	用物齐备，治疗车上下放置合理	4	一项不符扣 1 分	
	环境		环境符合要求	2	一项不符扣 2 分	
	患者	2	了解患者病情、合作程度、口腔和鼻腔情况及气管切开处	2	一项不符扣 1 分	
实施 70	核对解释	6	核对床号、姓名	2	一项不符扣 2 分	
			解释操作目的及配合方法	4	一项不符扣 2 分	
	吸痰前准备	8	检查患者口腔和鼻腔，有义齿者取下	4	一项不符扣 2 分	
			摆体位，患者头偏向一侧，面向护士	2	一项不符扣 2 分	
			置弯盘于患者口角旁	2	一项不符扣 2 分	
	吸痰	38	安装压力表，调至正确负压	4	一项不符扣 1 分	
			检查吸痰装置是否通畅	2	一项不符扣 2 分	
			检查并正确打开无菌缸盖	2	一项不符扣 2 分	
			检查吸痰管包装（名称、规格、有效期及有无漏气）	4	一项不符扣 1 分	
			为患者铺好治疗巾	2	一项不符扣 2 分	
			戴手套，正确取出吸痰管，包装袋放于污物桶内	6	一项不符扣 2 分	
			连接吸痰管	2	一项不符扣 2 分	
			试吸，检查吸痰管是否通畅	4	一项不符扣 2 分	
			吸痰（保证无负压插入，插入 10～15 cm，带负压旋转提拉，动作轻柔，时间少于 15 s）	6	一项不符扣 2 分	
			冲管，拔下吸痰管，连接管放置合理	4	一项不符扣 2 分	
			关压力表	2	一项不符扣 2 分	
	操作后整理	18	检查并正确取出纱布	2	一项不符扣 2 分	
			将连接管头端包好	2	一项不符扣 2 分	
			观察患者（面色、呼吸等），观察痰液颜色、性质及量等	6	一项不符扣 2 分	
			擦净脸部分泌物，撤去治疗巾	2	一项不符扣 2 分	
			为患者摆舒适体位	2	一项不符扣 2 分	
			整理用物，洗手并记录	4	一项不符扣 2 分	
评价 20	熟练	8	动作轻柔、熟练、步骤合理	2	一项不符扣 2 分	
			相关理论知识掌握熟练，遵守无菌原则	4	酌情扣分	
			按规定时间完成（5 min）	2	每超过 30 s 扣 1 分	
	效果	2	患者感觉安全舒适，无不良反应	2	酌情扣分	
	沟通	10	英语发音准确，语言流畅，关爱患者，沟通有效	10	酌情扣分	
主考教师：			日期：	总分：100	得分：	

评分标准：91～100 分为优，81～90 分为良，71～80 分为中，60～70 分为差，低于 60 分为不及格。

Chapter 7
Nasogastric Gavage
鼻　饲　法

7.1　Nasogastric Tube Insertion and Feeding
插胃管和鼻饲

Purpose　操作目的

To provide food or medications via nasogastric (NG) tubes for patients who are unable to take food by mouth in order to meet their needs of nutrition and treatments. This procedure is usually used for premature infants or patients who are unconscious, with oral disease or after oral operation, lockjaw, critical illness or tumor of upper alimentary canal.

对不能自行经口进食的患者以鼻饲管(简称胃管)供给食物或药物,以满足患者营养或治疗的需要,常用于早产儿或昏迷、口腔疾病或口腔手术后、破伤风、病情危重或上消化道肿瘤等患者。

Assessment　评估

1. Assess the patient's age, level of consciousness, health condition (capacity to swallow, functioning of the gastrointestinal tract, presence of nose or mouth disease, esophagus varicosity or obstruction, nutritional status), diagnosis and purpose of NG tube insertion and feeding.

评估患者的年龄、意识、病情(吞咽能力、胃肠道功能、有无鼻腔或口腔疾病、食管静脉曲张或食管梗阻、营养状况)、诊断、插胃管及鼻饲的目的。

2. Assess the status of nasal mucosa including swelling, bleeding or inflammation.

评估鼻腔黏膜情况,包括有无肿胀、出血或炎症等。

3. Assess the patency of nostril, noting the presence of deviated nasal septum or nasal polypus.

评估患者鼻道通畅情况,注意有无鼻中隔弯曲或鼻息肉等。

4. Assess the patient's psychological status, ability to cooperate, communication skills and understanding of NG tube insertion and feeding.

评估患者的心理状态、合作程度、表达能力、对插胃管及鼻饲的了解程度。

Gather equipment 物品准备

治疗盘内:feeding formula or medication solution(38～40 ℃)鼻饲液或药液(38～40 ℃), liquid paraffin 液体石蜡,swabs 棉签,adhesive tape 胶布,a glass of warm boiled water 一杯温开水, water thermometer 水温计,无菌鼻饲包(内备:sterile bowl 治疗碗,sterile nasogastric tube 消毒胃管(NG tube of appropriate size 规格合适的胃管),sterile forceps or sterile gloves 无菌镊子或无菌手套,curved forceps 血管钳,50 mL syringe 50 mL 注射器,tongue blade 压舌板,drapes 治疗巾,sterile gauze 无菌纱布)。

治疗盘外: prescription chart or treatment sheet 医嘱单或治疗单,kidney basin 弯盘,flashlight 手电筒,rubber band or clamp 橡胶圈或夹子,safety pin 别针,stethoscope 听诊器,hand sanitizer 洗手液。

Procedure 操作过程

1. Report and tidy your dress.

报告并整理仪表。

2. Check the validity of hand sanitizer and wash hands in 7 steps and put on the mask.

检查洗手液的有效期,7 步洗手法洗手并戴口罩。

3. Gather and check equipments. Check the type, amount and time of tube feeding against the prescription chart. Checking the expiration date of the feeding

formula and its temperature.

备齐并检查用物。根据医嘱核对鼻饲液的种类、量及鼻饲时间。检查鼻饲液的有效期及温度。

4. Wash hands and remove the mask.

洗手、摘口罩。

5. Assess the working environment.

评估操作环境。

6. Check the patient's bed number and name.

核对床头卡上床号和患者姓名。

7. Take the equipment to the bedside. Check the patient's name.

携用物至患者床旁。核对患者姓名。

8. Assess the patient's swallow.

评估患者吞咽能力。

9. Assist the patient to remove glasses and dentures.

协助患者取下眼镜及义齿。

10. Position the patient.

摆体位。

(1) Position a conscious patient in high Fowler's position or upright position. If the patient is unable to maintain upright position, assist him/her to right lateral position.

清醒患者取半坐位或坐位。如果患者无法坐起，则协助其取右侧卧位。

(2) Position an unconscious patient in supine position and remove the pillow with the head upward.

昏迷患者取去枕平卧位，头向后仰。

11. Wash hands and put on a mask.

洗手、戴口罩。

12. Place a cloth under the patient's chin and a basin within reach.

颌下铺治疗巾，将弯盘置于便于取用处。

13. Check the nostrils for patency and select one nostril with greater air flow without any mucous membrane damage or inflammation.

检查鼻腔是否通畅，选择较通畅、没有黏膜损伤或炎症的一侧鼻腔插管。

14. Clean the nostrils with swabs.

用棉签清洁鼻腔。

15. Determine the tube length to be inserted and mark with a piece of tape or oil

pen (the length for adults is 45-55 cm in general).

确定插管的长度并用小胶布或油性笔做标记(一般成人插入长度为 45～55 cm)。

(1) Measure the distance from the tip of the nose to the earlobe and then to the tip of the xiphoid process of the sternum.

测量从鼻尖经耳垂至胸骨剑突处的距离。

(2) Or measure the distance from the hair border on the forehead to the tip of the xiphoid process of the sternum.

或测量从前额发际至胸骨剑突处的距离。

16. Lubricate the tip and first few inches of the NG tube.

润滑胃管前端。

17. Let the patient know that the NG tube insertion is to begin.

告诉患者开始插胃管。

18. Hold the tip of the NG tube using sterile forceps or two hands wearing sterile gloves, insert the tube through the selected nostril gently.

用无菌镊子或戴无菌手套夹持胃管前端,沿选定的鼻腔轻轻插入胃管。

19. When the tube arrives at the throat (10-15 cm), insert the tube according to the patient's level of consciousness.

当插至咽喉部(10～15 cm)时,根据患者的意识状况进行插管。

(1) Encourage the conscious patient to dry swallow or swallow sips of water (unless contraindicated) to assist the tube insertion.

鼓励清醒患者做吞咽动作或饮少量水(除非禁忌),以助胃管插入。

(2) For unconscious patient, lift the head with one hand and make his/her chin touch the chest, insert the tube with the other hand.

对昏迷患者,一手托起患者头部,使其下颌靠近胸骨柄,用另一手插管。

20. Continue advancing the NG tube until the mark is reached. If it meets resistance, rotate the tube gently or have the patient open mouth and inspect oropharynx to be sure that the tube is not coiled in the back of the throat.

继续插入胃管至标记处。如遇阻力,轻轻旋转胃管或让患者张口,检查胃管是否卷曲在咽后壁。

21. Determine the tube is in the patient's stomach by one or more of the following methods.

使用以下一种或多种方法确认胃管是否在胃内。

(1) Attach the catheter-tip syringe to the free end of the NG tube and aspirate. If gastric fluid can be obtained, it means the tube is in the stomach.

胃管末端连接甘油注射器并回抽。如果能抽出胃液，说明胃管在胃内。

(2) If no gastric fluid can be obtained.

如果没有胃液抽出。

① Place the free end of the NG tube under water and ask the patient to take a deep breath. If on bubbles appear, it means the tube is not in the trachea.

将胃管末端置于水中，嘱患者深呼吸。若无气泡逸出，说明胃管没有进入气管。

② Inject 10 mL of air through the NG tube rapidly and listen with the stethoscope over the stomach. If a rush of air can be heard, it means the tube has reached the stomach.

置听诊器于患者胃部，快速经胃管向胃内注入 10 mL 空气。如能听到气过水声，说明胃管在胃内。

22. When the NG tube is confirmed to be in the stomach, remove the tape used to mark the tube length, tape the tube securely over the nose bridge and cheek in order to prevent tube migration.

证实胃管在胃内后，揭去标记长度用的胶布，用胶布固定胃管在患者鼻翼及颊部，以防胃管移位。

23. Before initiating tube feeding, check the gastric residual and then flush the tube with small amount of warm boiled water.

鼻饲前，检查胃残液量，然后用少量温开水冲洗胃管。

24. Fill a syringe with feeding formula or medication solution and attach it to the end of the NG tube, inject them slowly through the NG tube.

用注射器抽吸鼻饲液或药液，连接于胃管末端，并缓慢经胃管注入。

25. When disconnecting the syringe, pinch the free end of the NG tube to prevent air from going into the tube.

分离注射器时，反折胃管末端，避免空气进入胃管。

26. Refill and inject the feeding formula or medication solution until prescribed amount has been delivered to the patient.

再次抽吸并注入，直至全部鼻饲液或药液注完。

27. Flush the tube with small amount of warm boiled water once again to prevent tube obstruction by feeding formula.

再次用少量温开水冲洗胃管，以防胃管被鼻饲液堵塞。

28. Cover the free end of the NG tube with a piece of sterile gauze and fold it, loop a rubber band around the tube or clamp it, pin it to the patient's gown, leaving some degree of slack for head movement.

将胃管末端用无菌纱布包好并反折，用橡皮圈扎紧或用夹子夹紧，用别针固定胃管于患者衣服上，留下松动的空间以便患者头部转动。

29. Warn the patient not to pull out the NG tube and let him/her know the importance of tube securing.

提醒患者勿拔出胃管并告知胃管固定的重要性。

30. Explain the patient the necessary of tube flushing, right position and oral hygiene.

向患者讲解胃管冲洗、正确卧位及口腔护理的必要性。

31. Ask the patient to notify nurse immediately whenever any unusual effects are occurring.

告知患者如有不适立即告知护士。

32. Post-procedure 整理

(1) Provide oral and nasal hygiene if necessary.

必要时清洁患者口鼻。

(2) After tube feeding, have the patient remain the same position for at least 20 minutes and then adopt a comfortable position.

鼻饲后，让患者维持原卧位至少 20 min，然后取舒适卧位。

(3) Tidy up the patient's bed.

整理床单位。

(4) Wash and clean the used catheter-tip syringe, place it in the tray and cover it. The syringe should be changed everyday.

洗净鼻饲用的注射器，放于治疗盘内并盖好，每日更换一次。

(5) Discard other used equipment appropriately.

合理清理其他用物。

(6) Wash hands and remove the mask.

洗手、摘口罩。

(7) Sign the prescription chart or treatment sheet to indicate that the NG tube insertion and feeding has been administered.

在医嘱单或治疗单上签名，表示插胃管鼻饲已执行。

(8) Observe and record the patient's response including choking, respiratory distress, nausea, vomiting, abdominal distention or pain during and after tube feeding.

观察、记录鼻饲时及鼻饲后患者的反应，包括有无呛咳、呼吸困难、恶心、呕吐、腹胀或腹痛等。

(9) Record the type, amount and time of tube feeding, the volume and color of gastric residual.

记录鼻饲液的种类和量、鼻饲时间、胃残液量及颜色。

7.2 Discontinuing a Nasogastric Tube
拔出胃管

Gather equipment 物品准备

prescription chart or treatment sheet 医嘱单或治疗单，tray 治疗盘，curved / kidney basin 弯盘，gauze or tissues 纱布或纸巾，water for oral hygiene 漱口水，disposable gloves 一次性手套。

Procedure 操作过程

1. Verify doctor's order.

查阅医嘱。

2. Wash hands. Take the equipment to the patient's bedside.

洗手。携用物到患者床旁。

3. Identify the patient and assess his/her health condition.

确认患者并评估病情。

4. Explain to patient the reason for discontinuing the NG tube.

向患者解释拔除胃管的理由，指导患者如何配合。

5. Put on disposable gloves.

戴一次性手套。

6. If discontinuing a NG tube for GI decompression, disconnect the NG tube from the decompression unit and clamp the free end of the tube, then turn off the electrical suction equipment.

如果要拔除胃肠减压用的胃管，先将胃管与减压装置分离并夹紧胃管末端，然后关闭电动胃肠减压器。

7. Place a basin under the patient's chin. Unpin the NG tube from the patient's gown and remove the tap from his/her nose bridge and cheek.

置弯盘于患者颌下，取下患者衣服上固定胃管的别针，揭去鼻翼及颊部上的胶布。

8. Wrap the tube near the patient's nose with a piece of gauze or tissues, brush it while removing.

用纱布或纸巾包裹近鼻处的胃管,边拔边擦胃管。

(1) Method 1: Remove the tube slowly, when the NG tube will pass the throat, ask the patient to take a deep breath and hold breath, and remove the tube quickly.

方法一:慢慢拔管,当胃管将到咽喉时,嘱患者深吸气后屏气并快速拔出胃管。

(2) Method 2: Ask the patient to breath deeply, remove the tube when the patient is exhaling, remove it quickly when it will pass the throat.

方法二:嘱患者深呼吸,在患者呼气时拔管,到咽喉处快速拔出。

9. Place the tube in the basin or medical waste receiver, and then remove the basin.

将胃管放入弯盘或医用垃圾袋,然后撤离弯盘。

10. Inspect any erosion of nasal and oral mucous membranes due to pressure from the NG tube. Clean the patient's face and nares. Assist the patient to rinse the mouth and position him/her in comfortable position.

观察患者鼻腔、口腔黏膜有无因胃管压迫致损伤等。清洁患者面部及鼻孔。协助患者漱口并取舒适卧位。

11. Remove and dispose of gloves into medical waste receiver. Tidy up the bed, discard all used equipment appropriately, and wash hands.

脱下手套放入医用垃圾袋。整理床铺,合理清理用物,洗手。

12. Record the time of tube removal. Observe the patient for abdominal distention, nausea and vomiting.

记录拔管时间。观察患者有无腹胀、恶心、呕吐等。

Precautions for NG tube feeding 鼻饲的注意事项

1. Before initiating tube feeding each time, determine that the NG tube is properly located in the stomach and is patent. Flush the NG tube with some warm boiled water before tube feeding. Clean the tube with some warm boiled water once again after tube feeding in order to prevent metamorphosing of formula or obstruction with formula.

每次鼻饲前,应证实胃管在胃内且通畅,并用少量温开水冲洗胃管后再进行鼻饲。鼻饲完毕后再次用温开水冲洗胃管。以防鼻饲液积存于管腔变质或阻塞胃管。

2. Aspirate all gastric residual with a syringe and measure before tube feeding each time. Return the gastric contents immediately through the tube so as not to cause any fluid or electrolyte losses.

每次灌注食物前用注射器抽出胃内容物并测量胃残液量,并马上经胃管注回胃内防止水、电解质失衡。

3. Each tube feeding should not be over 200 mL at one time. The interval between feedings should be at least 2 hours and the temperature of the feeding formula should be maintained within 38-40 ℃.

每次鼻饲量不超过 200 mL。间隔时间应至少为 2 h。鼻饲液温度应保持在 38～40 ℃。

4. Tablets should be crushed (enteric coated is never crushed) and capsules should be opened. Dissolve the powder in some warm boiled water before administering medications via a NG tube.

药片应研碎(肠溶片不可),胶囊应打开。用温开水溶解药粉后经胃管给药。

5. When disconnecting syringe, pinch the free end of the tube to prevent air from gong into the NG tube and causing abdominal distention.

每次分离注射器时应反折胃管末端,避免灌入空气引起腹胀。

6. Have the patient remain the same position for at least 20 minutes after tube feeding. Upright position can minimize risk for backflow and prevent aspiration in case vomiting occurs. Do not elevate the head of the bed for patients with spinal injury.

鼻饲后让患者保持原卧位至少 20 min,坐位能减少胃液反流及防止呕吐物误吸。脊柱损伤者不宜抬高床头。

7. If the patient is receiving tube feeding for a long period of time, provide the patient with oral hygiene twice a day and change the NG tube at regular intervals.

长期鼻饲者应每日进行空腔护理两次,并定期更换胃管。

8. Never administer NG tube feeding for patients with esophagus varicosity or obstruction.

食管静脉曲张或食管梗阻的患者禁忌使用鼻饲法。

New Words and Expressions
单 词 表

nasogastric [neizəu'gæstrik] *adj.* 鼻饲的

premature ['premətʃə] *adj.* 早产的;不成熟的;比预期早的

unconscious [ʌn'kɔnʃəs] *adj.* 无意识的;失去知觉的;不省人事的

lockjaw ['lɔkdʒɔː] *n.* 破伤风;[医] 牙关紧闭症

tumor ['tjuːmə] *n.* 肿瘤;肿块

alimentary [ˌæli'mentəri] *adj.* 食物的

swallow [ˈswɔləu] *vi*. 吞下;咽下

gastrointestinal [ˌgæstrəuinˈtestinl] *adj*. 胃肠的

esophagus [iːˈsɔfəgəs] *n*. 食管;食道

varicosity [ˌværiˈkɔsiti] *n*. 静脉曲张;静脉瘤

obstruction [əbˈstrʌkʃən] *n*. 障碍;阻碍

diagnosis [ˌdaiəgˈnəusis] *n*. 诊断

nasal [ˈneizəl] *adj*. 鼻的;鼻音的

mucosa [mjuːˈkəusə] *n*. 黏膜

inflammation [infləˈmeiʃən] *n*. 炎症

patency [ˈpeitənsi] *n*. 开放

nostril [ˈnɔstril] *n*. 鼻孔

deviated [ˈdiːvieitid] *vt*. 使偏离

septum [ˈseptəm] *n*. 隔膜

polypus [ˈpɔlipəs] *n*. 息肉

psychological [saikəˈlɔdʒikəl] *adj*. 心理的;精神上的

formula [ˈfɔːmjulə] *n*. 配方

prescription [prisˈkripʃən] *n*. 药方;指示

expiration [ˌekspaiəˈreiʃən] *n*. 呼气

lateral [ˈlætərəl] *adj*. 侧面的

supine [sjuːˈpain] *adj*. 仰卧的

chin [tʃin] *n*. 下巴

mucous [ˈmjuːkəs] *adj*. 黏液的;分泌黏液的

membrane [ˈmembrein] *n*. 膜

earlobe [ˈiələub] *n*. 耳垂

xiphoid [ˈzifɔid] *n*. 剑状突起;剑状

sternum [ˈstəːnəm] *n*. 胸骨

lubricate [ˈluːbrikeit] *vt*. 使……润滑;给……加润滑油

contraindicated [kɔntrəˈindikeitid] *vt*. 禁忌(某种疗法或药物)

rotate [rəuˈteit] *vt*. 使旋转;使转动;使轮流

oropharynx [ˌɔːrəuˈfæriŋks] *n*. 口咽

coiled [kɔild] *v*. 卷(coil 的过去式和过去分词);盘绕

syringe [ˈsirindʒ] *n*. 注射器

aspirate [ˈæspireit] *vt*. 吸入

gastric [ˈgæstrik] *adj*. 胃的;胃部的

trachea [trəˈkiə] *n.* 气管

securely [siˈkjuəli] *adv.* 安全地;牢固地

migration [maiˈgreiʃən] *n.* 移动

residual [riˈzidjuəl] *n.* 剩余;残渣

flush [flʌʃ] *vt.* 用水冲洗

slack [slæk] *adj.* 松弛的;*vi.* 松懈

hygiene [ˈhaidʒiːn] *n.* 卫生

choking [ˈtʃəukiŋ] *v.* 阻塞;使……窒息(choke 的 ing 形式)

nausea [ˈnɔːsjə] *n.* 恶心

distention [disˈtenʃn] *n.* 膨胀

decompression [diːkəmˈpreʃn] *n.* 解压;降压

exhaling [ˈeksheiliŋ] *v.* 呼气;发散

erosion [iˈrəuʒn] *n.* 侵蚀,腐蚀

nares [ˈneiriːz] *n.* 鼻孔(naris 的复数)

Communication Model
沟 通 模 板

Self-introduction Model 常规介绍模板

Good morning/afternoon teachers, my name is ××, I come from class ××, my student's number is ××. Today, I am going to show you the process of nasogastric gavage, the equipments I have prepared are... ,everything is ready, may I start?

老师上午/下午好,我是××,来自××班,我的学号是××。今天我要展示的操作是鼻饲术,所准备的用物有……,准备完毕,请求开始。

Assessment 评估

The ward is tidy and well ventilated. There is no cleaning half an hour ago. The surgical incision of the patient is in the mouth, so he can't eat food or medicine through the mouth. The patient is in good mental state, and swallowing reflex is normal, he can cooperate with me.

病室整洁、通风良好。半小时前无人打扫房间。患者口腔有外伤伤口,他不能经口

进食或服药。患者精神状态良好,吞咽反射正常,有配合能力。

Communication 沟通

Good morning, sir. I am your nurse today. You can call me ××. Would you tell me your full name please? OK. Mr ××, how do you feel now? How was your sleep last night? Do you have pain of the incision site? (Patient: Yes, I feel a kind of swollen with a little bit of pain in the mouth.)

早上好先生,我是您今天的责任护士,你可以叫我××。能告诉我您的名字吗?好,××先生,您现在感觉怎么样? 昨晚睡得好吗? 您口腔的伤口还疼痛吗?(患者:我感觉嘴里还有些肿胀和疼痛。)

Don't worry. This is your first day after the operation. It is normal to experience the feelings that you have described. Because your incision in the mouth, you can not eat through the mouth for a while. In order for you to intake enough nutrition and fluid, we need to put a nasogastric tube through your nose into the stomach so that we can give you the nutrition and liquid through the tube. Please cooperate with me during the procedure. Have you had the experience of a nasogastric tube being placed into your stomach? (Patient: No.)

别担心。在手术后的第一天这些感受是很正常的。因为您口腔中有手术切口,您在一段时间都不能经口进食。为了您能够正常摄入足够的营养和液体,我需要帮您从鼻腔插入一根鼻胃管到胃内来灌注流质饮食。请在操作中配合我做吞咽动作。您以前有过下鼻胃管的经历吗?(患者:没有。)

You might feel some sense of nausea during the procedure, you may take deep breath to reduce the discomfort and swallow the tube at the same time. Don't worry, It dose not be hurt.

你会在插管过程中感觉到恶心的感觉,请深呼吸来减轻这种不适感并同时做吞咽动作。不用担心,插管并不疼。

Good. This procedure may take up to 10 minutes. Do you need to go to the restroom now? (Patient: Not now. Thank you!)

很好,操作过程可能会持续 10 min,你需要现在先去下卫生间吗?(患者:现在不用。谢谢!)

Positioning(upright position) 取体位

OK, I will raise the head of the bed.

好,现在我将为您摇起床头。

Place a drape and kidney basin, checking nostrils 铺巾置弯盘，检查鼻腔

Are you having a stuffy nose or some other discomforts now? Can I check your nose and mouth? Do you normally have problem with swallowing or history of throwing up (or vomiting) after meals? I am going to clean the nostril now. You will feel a little cold.

您有鼻塞或其他不适吗？让我来检查下您的鼻腔和口腔状况。您通常在进餐时或饭后会有吞咽困难或呕吐的问题吗？我要为您清洁下鼻腔，您可能会觉得有些凉。

Marking the tube 标记胃管

Now I am going to insert the nasogastric tube. You may take slow and deep breaths if you feel nausea. Please let me know if there are any other discomforts.

现在我要为您插管了，请您缓慢的深呼吸，如果有其他不适请示意我。

Inserting the tube 插管

I am putting the tube in now. Please relax. Very good, it has already passed the throat. Please swallow now, very good. Please open your mouth and let me check the tube. It is good. You have done a great job. Now it is in the right place. Are you OK? (Patient: I feel like something blocking in my throat.)

现在管已经进入咽喉了，请放松，很好，管顺利地通过了咽喉部。请做吞咽动作，很棒！张开嘴让我查看一下下管情况，非常好，您真的很棒！管已经在指定的位置了，您感觉还好吗？（患者：我感觉咽喉有异物感。）

That is OK. It is a normal feeling caused by the tube. You may continue deep breaths, and you will get used to it in a little while. I am going to confirm the position and fix the tube. (Patient: All right.)

没关系，那是因为管在咽喉处产生的正常感觉，你只要持续地深呼吸，一会就会适应的。我现在需要确定胃管的位置并固定胃管。（患者：好的。）

Well done. Now I am going to infuse the liquid through the tube to your stomach to get the nutrition your body needed. Please let me know if you have any discomforts while I do the tube feeding.

很好，现在我要通过胃管为您灌注流质饮食来为您提供身体所需的营养。在喂食过程中有任何不适请告诉我。

Now I have already finished, how do you feel? (Patient: Nothing particular.)

完成了，您感觉怎么样？（患者：没什么特别的。）

That is good. This tube needs to be in for a period of time till your oral wound is healed. Please be careful not to pull it out when you get up or turn from side to side. Nurses are going to help you cleaning the mouth regularly too. Please report whenever you have abdominal pain or other discomforts, we will come to check regularly. Please remain this upright position for 30 minutes and have a good rest. Hope you recover soon! I am leaving now. Please press the call signal if you need us. We will come to see you as soon as possible.

很好，这根管需要您留置一段时间直到口腔伤口愈合，请在起床或翻身时注意不要将管拔出。护士会为您常规做口腔护理的。当您出现腹痛或其他不适我们会过来为您做检查。请维持这个体位 30 min，好好休息。祝您早日康复。有什么问题按呼叫器找我，我会尽快过来帮助您。

Scoring Criteria 10
评分细则 10

项目		总分	技术操作要求	标准分	扣分说明	得分
评估 12	仪表	4	仪表端庄、服装整洁、修剪指甲、洗手、戴口罩	4	一项不符扣 2 分	
	物品	4	用物齐备、治疗车上下放置合理	2	一项不符扣 2 分	
	准备		环境符合要求	2	一项不符扣 2 分	
	患者	4	了解患者诊断、意识状态、合作程度、身体状况	2	一项不符扣 1 分	
			鼻饲液、鼻腔状况	2	一项不符扣 1 分	
实施 68	核对	4	核对床号、姓名	2	一项不符扣 1 分	
			解释内容合理(操作目的、配合方法及注意事项)	2	一项不符扣 2 分	
	插管	36	安置体位正确、恰当(表述清醒和昏迷患者体位)	4	一项不符扣 2 分	
			颌下铺治疗巾,找剑突做标记,放弯盘	4	一项不符扣 2 分	
			检查鼻腔并清洁鼻腔	2	一项不符扣 2 分	
			正确测量胃管插入长度(口述两种方法)	4	一项不符扣 2 分	
			润滑胃管前端(10～15 cm)	2	一项不符扣 2 分	
			插管正确(动作轻柔、无污染,保持胃管清洁)	2	一项不符扣 2 分	
			插至 10～15 cm 时,使患者配合(清醒及昏迷)	4	一项不符扣 2 分	
			正确处理插管中出现的情况(恶心、咳嗽、呼吸困难、发绀及插入困难)	6	一项不符扣 2 分	
			能准确施行 3 种判断胃管在胃内的方法	6	一项不符扣 2 分	
			胃管固定牢固、美观	2	一项不符扣 2 分	
	灌注食物	15	回抽胃液,判断胃管是否在胃内,弃去胃液并清洗注射器	4	一项不符扣 2 分	
			灌入少量温开水	2	一项不符扣 2 分	
			灌食(鼻饲液的量、温度、速度适宜,反折胃管,避免空气进入)	2	一项不符扣 2 分	
			操作过程中注意观察患者反应	1	一项不符扣 1 分	
			灌完食物后再灌入少量温开水冲管	2	一项不符扣 2 分	
			正确处理胃管末端(反折,纱布包好)	2	一项不符扣 2 分	
			妥善安置患者(清洁口鼻,维持原卧位 30 min)	2	一项不符扣 2 分	
	拔管	8	夹紧胃管末端、置治疗巾、弯盘于颌下	4	一项不符扣 2 分	
			拔管手法正确、指导配合正确	2	一项不符扣 2 分	
			擦拭面部、胶布痕迹	2	一项不符扣 2 分	
	整理	5	患者卧位舒适、衣物整洁,床单位整洁	2	一项不符扣 2 分	
			用物处理正确,洗手、记录	3	一项不符扣 1 分	

续表

项目		总分	技术操作要求	标准分	扣分说明	得分
评价 20	熟练	8	动作熟练,步骤合理,无菌观念强	4	一项不符扣 2 分	
			掌握相关知识,15 min 完成	4	每过 30 s 扣 1 分	
	效果	2	患者感觉舒适安全、无不良反应	2	酌情扣分	
	沟通	10	发音准确,语言流畅,关爱患者,有效沟通	10	酌情扣分	
主考教师:			日期:	总分:100	得分:	

评分标准:91～100 分为优,81～90 分为良,71～80 分为中,60～70 分为差,低于 60 分为不及格。

Chapter 8
Urinary Catheterization
导 尿 术

8.1 Retention Catheterization
留置导尿管

Purpose 操作目的

1. To monitor the output of a critically ill patient or patient in shock by recording the amount of urine per hour and measuring the specific gravity of urine accurately.

对于危重、休克患者，准确记录每小时尿量、测量尿比重，以密切观察患者的病情变化。

2. To allow the bladder to empty fully and continuously in order to prevent accidental bladder injury during pelvic surgery.

为盆腔手术患者排空膀胱，使膀胱保持空虚，避免手术中误伤。

3. Retaining a catheter for postoperative patients with urologic diseases can provide continuous urinary bladder drainage or irrigation. This will reduce tension on the surgical incision and facilitate its healing.

为泌尿系统疾病手术后的患者留置导尿管，便于引流或冲洗，并可减轻手术切口的张力，有利于切口的愈合。

4. To maintain a continuous outflow of urine for incontinent patients or patients with perineal incision in order to keep the perineum area clean and dry.

为尿失禁或会阴部有伤口的患者持续引流尿液，以保持会阴部清洁干燥。

5. To provide bladder functional training for incontinent patients.

为尿失禁患者进行膀胱功能训练。

Assessment 评估

1. Assess the patient's gender, age, level of consciousness, health condition, diagnosis and purpose of retention catheterization.

评估患者的性别、年龄、意识、病情、诊断及留置导尿管的目的。

2. Assess the patient's urinary elimination, bladder fullness, the condition of perineal skin and mucosa, etc.

评估患者的排尿状况、膀胱充盈度及会阴部皮肤黏稠情况等。

3. Assess the patient's psychological status, ability to cooperate, communication skills, self-care ability, and understanding of retention catheterization.

评估患者的心理状态、合作程度、表达能力、自理能力及对留置导尿管术的了解程度。

Equipment preparation 用物准备

无菌导尿包(治疗巾上层备): equipment for disinfecting the perineum preliminarily 外阴初步消毒用物: sterile balls 消毒棉球, forceps 镊子, kidney basin 弯盘, 1 sterile rubber glove 无菌橡胶手套 1 只, gauzes 纱布。

无菌导尿包(治疗巾里备): kidney basins 弯盘, urinary catheter 尿管, 4 cotton balls 4 个棉球, forceps 镊子, curved forceps 弯止血钳, lubricant cotton balls 润滑油棉球, specimen bottle 标本瓶, urine bag 集尿袋带别针, syringe 注射器, fenestrated drape 一次性洞巾, sterile rubber gloves 无菌橡胶手套, gauzes 纱布。

其他: sterile transfer forceps 无菌持物钳和钳筒一套, drape 垫巾, kidney basin 弯盘, bath towel 浴巾, bedpan 便盆及 toilet wipes 便器巾。

Procedure 操作流程

Male Retention Catheterization 男性留置导尿术

1. Report and tidy your dress.

报告并整理仪表。

2. Check the validity of hand sanitizer and wash hands in 7 steps and put on the

mask.

检查洗手液的有效期，7 步洗手法洗手并戴口罩。

3. Gather equipments and check for the prescription and equipments.

备齐用物，核对医嘱及用品。

4. Wash hands and remove the mask.

洗手、摘口罩。

5. Take the equipment to the ward. Assess the working environment, close the doors and windows and provide the privacy environment to the patient.

携用物至病室内。评估操作环境，关闭门窗，为患者提供隐私环境。

6. Check the patient's bed number and name.

核对床头卡上床号和患者姓名。

7. Take the equipment to the bedside. Check the patient's name. Explain the purpose and procedure of the operation, and get cooperation from the patient.

携用物至患者床旁。核对患者姓名。解释操作目的和过程，与患者取得合作。

8. Assist the patient to take off the opposite trouser and use it to cover the near side leg. Cover the opposite leg with a quilt.

协助患者脱去对侧裤腿并盖在近侧腿上，用盖被遮盖对侧腿。

9. Assist the patient to supine position with knees flexed and thighs externally rotated, leaving only the perineum exposed.

协助患者取仰卧位，两腿屈膝、外展，只暴露外阴。

10. Place a disposable cloth under the buttocks.

将一次性治疗巾铺于臀下。

11. Open the cover of the waste bin, wash hands and put on the mask.

打开污桶盖，洗手、戴口罩。

12. Disinfecting the perineum. Place a basin near the perineum and open the urethral catheterization bag, place the bowl (containing cotton balls and forceps) between the patient's thighs. Wear disposable gloves.

会阴初步消毒。将弯盘放于外阴旁，打开导尿包，取出初步消毒盘(内盛无菌手套、碘伏、消毒棉球、纱布和镊子)置于患者两腿间，戴手套。

13. Wear the gloves and take out the forceps to pick up the cotton balls into the sterile tray, disinfecting the perineum.

用戴手套的手取出无菌镊子，夹取消毒棉球于无菌盘内，消毒外阴。

14. Disinfect the monspubis first and then the penis and scrotum. With the other hand, hold the penis with a piece of gauze and retract foreskin to expose coronary

sulcus. Disinfect the meatus, glans and then coronary sulcus in a circular motion.

先消毒阴阜，消毒阴茎正面，另一手用无菌方纱裹住阴茎抬起，消毒阴茎背面、阴囊部；将包皮向后推暴露冠状沟，以尿道口为中心向外旋转擦拭尿道口、龟头至冠状沟。

15. Use a clean cotton ball for each wipe and place the used cotton balls in the basin.

每个棉球只用一次，用后放入弯盘内。

16. Move the bowl and basin to the end of the bed, remove the used gloves.

将治疗碗及弯盘移于床尾，摘手套。

17. Place a sterile urethral catheterization package between the patient's thighs. Open the package using aseptic techniques.

置导尿包于患者两腿之间。按无菌技术操作打开导尿包形成无菌区。

18. Wear sterile gloves, apply a sterile fenestrated drape over the patient's perineal area. Place the kidney basin near the perineal area and put the sterilized cotton ball into the kidney basin.

戴无菌手套，铺洞巾于患者会阴部。置弯盘于近会阴部，将消毒棉球倒入弯盘内。

19. Check the patency of the urinary catheter, and the integrity of the catheter balloon. Lubricate the tip and first few inches of the catheter with lubricated cotton balls and place the catheter in the basin. Attach the catheter to the drainage bag.

检查导尿管是否通畅，注水测试气囊是否完整。用蘸有润滑油的棉球润滑导尿管前段并置于弯盘内，连接集尿袋。

20. With one hand, grasp the penis with a piece of gauze and retract the foreskin to expose urethral meatus and maintain the hand in this position throughout the remainder of the procedure in order to prevent contamination of meatus.

一手用纱布裹住阴茎将包皮向后推，暴露尿道口、冠状沟，该手固定阴茎不动，以防污染尿道口。

21. With the other hand, pick up a cotton ball soaked with antiseptic solution using hemostat forceps and disinfect the meatus, glans and then coronary sulcus 3 times. Place the used cotton balls and forceps in a sterile basin and remove them to the foot of the bed.

另一手用镊子夹取消毒棉球，再次消毒，由尿道口向外旋转消毒龟头、冠状沟 3 次，最后用一个棉球消毒尿道口。消毒完毕，将使用过的消毒棉球和镊子放入弯盘内，移至床尾。

22. Place the other sterile basin containing a catheter beside the fenestra of the fenestrated drape. Ask the patient to take deep breaths.

将盛导尿管的无菌弯盘置于洞巾孔处，嘱患者深呼吸。

23. Insert the catheter through the meatus and then lift the penis 60° angle towards the patient's abdominal wall. Insert the catheter into the urethra about 20-22 cm in an adult or until urine flows out the catheter end. When urine appears, advance the catheter another 7～10 cm to ensure the balloon of the catheter is in the bladder.

提起阴茎与腹壁成60°角，将导尿管轻轻插入尿道20～22 cm或直至尿液流出。见尿后再插入7～10 cm，以确保导尿管的气囊在膀胱内。

24. Inflate the balloon with the exact amount of sterile water or sterile normal saline indicated on the catheter.

持注射器根据导管上注明的气囊容积向气囊内注入等量无菌水或无菌生理盐水。

25. Retract the catheter until you feel resistance. This indicates that the catheter tip is anchored in place above the bladder outlet.

轻拉到尿管有阻力感，即证实导尿管前端固定于膀胱口内。

26. Remove the fenestrated drape. Attach the end of the catheter to the tube of the drainage bag, fasten the tube to the bedsheet with a pin. Open the catheter.

撤去洞巾，将集尿袋用别针固定在床单上。开放导尿管。

27. Dry the patient's perineum, remove gloves and put the used catheterization package under the cart. Using a piece of adhesive tape fixed the cather and write down the time of retaining the urinary catheter. Assist the patient to put on pants, remove the disposable cloth and positioning.

擦拭患者外阴部，脱下手套，撤去导尿包放于治疗车下层。用一小条胶布固定导尿管并写下下管时间。帮助患者穿好裤子，撤治疗巾，使其保持舒适体位。

28. Wash hands again and take off the mask, providing health education to the patient.

洗手，摘口罩，健康宣教。

29. Tell the patient that perineal hygiene should be performed 1-2 times per day to keep the perineum clean.

告诉患者每天要进行1～2次会阴护理，以保持外阴清洁。

30. Encourage oral fluids (unless contraindicated) and introduce relative knowledge about the illness to the patient.

鼓励患者多喝水(除非禁忌)，并向患者介绍疾病相关知识。

31. Instruct the patient to keep the continuous-drainage bag below the level of the bladder and avoid compressing the bag in order to prevent backflow of urine.

指导患者集尿袋不要超过膀胱高度并避免挤压，防止尿液排出。

32. Instruct the patient to avoid pulling the catheter in order to avoid dislodging while turning in bed. Furthermore, the catheter should not be pressed or kinked.

指导患者翻身时勿牵拉以防导尿管脱出,注意导尿管不可受压或扭曲。

33. Open the curtain and windows.

拉开围帘,开窗。

34. Record the time of retaining the urinary catheter. Observe and record the amount, color, clarity, odor of urine, and the patient's response.

记录留置导尿管的时间,观察并记录尿液量、颜色、澄清度、气味及患者反应。

35. Post procedure.

整理用物。

Female Retention Catheterization 女性留置导尿术

1. Report and tidy your dress.

报告并整理仪表。

2. Check the validity of hand sanitizer and wash hands in 7 steps and put on the mask.

检查洗手液的有效期,7 步洗手法洗手并戴口罩。

3. Gather equipments and check for the prescription and equipments.

备齐用物,核对医嘱及用品。

4. Wash hands and remove the mask.

洗手、摘口罩。

5. Take the equipment to the ward. Assess the working environment, close the doors and windows and provide the privacy environment to the patient.

携用物至病室内。评估操作环境,关闭门窗,为患者提供隐私环境。

6. Check the patient's bed number and name.

核对床头卡上床号和患者姓名。

7. Take the equipment to the bedside. Check the patient's name. Explain the purpose and procedure of the operation, and get cooperation from the patient.

携用物至患者床旁。核对患者姓名。解释操作目的和过程,与患者取得合作。

8. Assist the patient take off the opposite trouser and use it to cover the near side leg, cover the opposite leg with a quilt.

协助患者脱去对侧裤腿并盖在近侧腿上,用盖被遮盖对侧腿。

9. Assist the patient to supine position with knees flexed and thighs externally rotated, leaving only the perineum exposed.

协助患者取仰卧位,两腿屈膝、外展,只暴露外阴。

10. Place a disposable cloth under the buttocks.

将一次性治疗巾铺于臀下。

11. Open the cover of the Waste bin, wash hands and put on the mask.

开污桶盖，洗手、戴口罩。

12. Place a basin near the perineum and open the urethral catheterization bag, place the bowl (containing cotton balls and forceps) between the patient's thighs. Wear disposable gloves.

将弯盘放于外阴旁，打开导尿包，取出初步消毒盘(内盛无菌手套、碘伏消毒棉球、纱布和镊子)置于患者两腿间，戴手套。

13. Open the bag of sterile cotton balls, wear the gloves and take out the forceps to pick up the cotton balls into the sterile tray, disinfecting the perineum.

打开消毒棉球包，用戴手套的手取出无菌镊子夹取消毒棉球于无菌盘内，消毒外阴。

14. With one hand, pick up a cotton ball soaked with antiseptic solution using hemostat forceps and disinfect the perineum orderly from outside to inside and from top to bottom. Disinfect the monspubis first and then the labia majors. Separate the labia majors with the other hand, disinfect the labia minora and then urethral meatus. Use a clean cotton ball for each wipe and place the used cotton balls in the basin.

一手用止血钳夹取消毒液棉球，按由外向内、自上而下的顺序消毒外阴。先消毒阴阜、大阴唇；另一手分开大阴唇，消毒小阴唇、尿道口。每个棉球只用一次，用后放进弯盘内。

15. Remove the bowl and basin, remove the used gloves.

撤走治疗碗和弯盘，脱下手套。

16. Place a sterile catheterization package between the patient's thighs. Open the package using aseptic techniques, keeping the equipment sterile.

置无菌包于患者两腿之间。按无菌技术操作打开导尿包，保持包内物品无菌。

17. Wear sterile gloves, apply a sterile fenestrated drape over the patient's perineal area. Place the kidney basin near the perineal area and put the sterilized cotton ball into the kidney basin.

戴无菌手套，铺洞巾于患者会阴部。置弯盘于近会阴部，将消毒棉球倒入弯盘内。

18. Check the patency of the urinary catheter, and the integrity of the catheter balloon. Lubricate the tip and first few inches of the catheter with lubricated cotton balls and place the catheter in the basin. Attach the catheter to the drainage bag.

检查导尿管是否通畅，注水测试气囊是否完整。用蘸有润滑油的棉球润滑导尿管前段并置于弯盘内，连接集尿袋。

19. With one hand, retract the labia minora to fully expose urethral meatus and maintain the hand in this position throughout the remainder of the procedure in order to prevent contamination of meatus.

一手分开并固定小阴唇，充分暴露尿道口，该手固定不动，以防污染尿道口。

20. With the other hand, pick up a cotton ball soaked with antiseptic solution using hemostat forceps and disinfect the meatus, labia minora and then meatus respectively. Place the used cotton balls and forceps in a sterile basin and remove them to the foot of the bed.

另一手用止血钳夹取消毒棉球，分别消毒尿道口、小阴唇、尿道口。棉球、止血钳用过后放入无菌弯盘内，然后撤至床尾。

21. Place the other sterile basin containing a catheter beside the fenestra of the fenestrated drape. Ask the patient to take deep breaths.

将盛导尿管的无菌弯盘置于洞巾孔处，嘱患者深呼吸。

22. Insert the catheter through the meatus into the urethra about 4-6 cm in an adult or until urine flows out the catheter end. When urine appears, advance the catheter another 7-10 cm to ensure the balloon of the catheter is in the bladder.

将导尿管从尿道口轻轻插入尿道 4～6 cm 或直至尿液流出。见尿液流后再插入 7～10 cm，以确保导尿管的气囊在膀胱内。

23. Release the labia minora and hold the catheter securely.

松开固定小阴唇的手以固定导尿管。

24. Inflate the balloon with the exact amount of sterile water or sterile normal saline indicated on the catheter.

持注射器根据导管上注明的气囊容积向气囊内注入等量无菌水或无菌生理盐水。

25. Retract the catheter until you feel resistance. This indicates that the catheter tip is anchored in place above the bladder outlet.

轻拉到尿管有阻力感，即证实导尿管前端固定于膀胱口内。

26. Remove the fenestrated drape. Attach the end of the catheter to the tube of the drainage bag, fasten the tube to the bedsheet with a pin. Open the catheter.

撤去洞巾，将集尿袋用别针固定在床单上，开放导尿管。

27. Dry the patient's perineum, remove gloves and put the used catheterization package under the cart. Using a piece of adhesive tape fixed the cathter and write down the time of retaining the urinary catheter. Assist the patient to put on pants, remove the disposable cloth and positioning.

擦拭患者外阴部，脱下手套，撤去导尿包放于治疗车下层。用一小条胶布固定导尿管并写下下管时间。帮助患者穿好裤子，撤去治疗巾，使其保持舒适体位。

28. Wash hands again and take off the mask, providing health education to the patient.

洗手、摘口罩，健康宣教。

29. Tell the patient that perineal hygiene should be performed 1-2 times per day to keep the perineum clean.

告诉患者每天要进行1～2次会阴护理，以保持外阴清洁。

30. Encourage oral fluids (unless contraindicated) and introduce relative knowledge about the illness to the patient.

鼓励患者多喝水(除非禁忌)，并向患者介绍疾病相关知识。

31. Instruct the patient to keep the continuous-drainage bag below the level of the bladder and avoid compressing the bag in order to prevent backflow of urine.

指导患者集尿袋不要超过膀胱高度并避免挤压，防止尿液溢出。

32. Instruct the patient to avoid pulling the catheter in order to avoid dislodging while turning in bed. Furthermore, the catheter should not be pressed or kinked.

指导患者翻身时勿牵拉以防导尿管脱出，且导尿管不可受压或扭曲。

33. Open the curtain and windows.

拉开围帘、开窗。

34. Record the time of retaining the urinary catheter. Observe and record the amount, color, clarity, odor of urine, and the patient's response.

记录留置导尿管的时间。观察并记录尿液量、颜色、澄清度、气味及患者反应。

35. Post procedure.

整理用物。

Nurse Alert 护理事项

1. Follow the checking procedure and use aseptic techniques strictly.

严格执行查对制度和无菌技术操作原则。

2. Ensure the patient's privacy and keep the patient warm by appropriate measures during the procedure.

操作过程中注意保护患者隐私，并采取适当的措施为患者保暖。

3. Identify the urethral meatus before inserting a catheter for female patient. An older female patient's urethral meatus always retracts, pay much more attention to

identify the meatus before inserting a catheter. If the catheter is mistakenly introduced into the patient's vagina, use a new sterile catheter and place it in urethra.

为女性患者插导尿管时，应准确辨别尿道口。老年女性尿道口回缩，插管时应细心辨别。若导尿管误插入阴道口，应更换无菌导尿管重新插入。

4. Be familiar with the anatomical characteristics of male and female urethra. Preform the procedure gently to avoid urethral injury.

应熟悉男性、女性尿道的解剖特点，动作轻稳，避免损伤患者尿道。

5. For a fragile patient with a fully distended bladder, do not empty more than 1000 mL of urine at the beginning in order to avoid fainting and hematuria.

对膀胱高度膨胀而极度衰弱的患者，第一次放尿不得超过 1000 mL，避免患者发生虚脱和血尿。

New Words and Expressions
单 词 表

catheterization [ˌkæθitəri'zeiʃn] *n.* [外科] 导管插入
bladder ['blædə] *n.* 膀胱；囊状物，可充气的囊袋
perineum [ˌperi'niːəm] *n.* [解剖]会阴
meatus [mi'eitəs] *n.* [解剖]道；[解剖]口；导管
urethra [juə'riːθrə] *n.* [解剖]尿道
labia minora *n.* [解剖]小阴唇

Communication model
沟 通 模 板

Self-introduction Model 常规介绍模板

Good morning/afternoon teachers, my name is ××, I come from class ××, my student's number is ××. Today, I am going to show you the process of urinary catheterization, the equipments I have prepared are..., everything is ready, may I start?

老师上午/下午好，我是××，来自××班，我的学号是××。今天我要展示的操作是导尿术，所准备的用物有……，准备完毕，请求开始。

Assessment 评估

The patient is in good psychological status. The patient with full bladder can understand the purpose of retention catheterization and he/she have the ability to cooperate with me.

患者精神状态良好，患者膀胱胀满，能够理解留置导尿管的目的并具有配合能力。

Communication 沟通

Good morning, sir. I'm your primary nurse, my name is ××. Would you tell me your full name? According to the doctor's order, I will do urinary catheteriztion for you to relieve your urine retention. I will insert a catheter to your bladder through your urethra, urine will come out through the catheter and you will feel much better afterwards. Let me exam your bladder and perineal skin condition. Yes, your bladder is very full due to the large amount of urine inside.

早上好，我是您的责任护士，我叫××，能告诉我您的名字吗？根据医嘱我要为您做留置导尿管来缓解您尿潴留的不适。导尿就是通过尿道插入导尿管至膀胱，尿液就会顺着导尿管流出到尿袋内，操作后您会感觉舒适些。让我来检查下您膀胱和会阴部皮肤的状况。您的膀胱高度胀满，里面充满了大量的尿液。

Now, I will take off your trousers, please flex your knees.

现在，我帮您脱下对侧的裤腿，请弯曲膝盖。

Please elevate buttocks.

请抬臀。

Now, I will clean the skin for you, don't be nervous, you will just feel a little cold.

现在我要为您消毒皮肤了，不要紧张，您只会感觉有些凉。

Do you feel cold? I have to clean your skin one more time.

您感觉冷吗？我还得再消毒一遍。

I will insert the catheter for you, please don't be nervous, breath deeply and relax.

现在我要为您插管了，请不要紧张，深呼吸并放松。

OK, it is done, the urine outflow from your bladder, do you feel much better? There are something you must know. First, drinking more water everyday is good for your condition and prevent infection. Second, to keep your perineum clean, nurses will performed perineal hygiene 1-2 times per day for you. Please keep the continuous-drainage bag below the level of the bladder and avoid compressing the bag in order to prevent backflow of urine. Last, avoid pulling the catheter while turning in bed and the catheter should not be pressed or kinked.

好，现在操作已经完成了，尿液已经从膀胱流出，您感觉好些了吗？有些事情您必须要知道。第一，每天多喝水对您的疾病和预防感染非常有利。第二，为保持您会阴的清洁，护士会每天为您做 1～2 次会阴护理。为防止尿液反流请不要将尿袋抬高超过膀胱的高度和避免挤压尿袋。最后，在翻身时不要牵拉尿管，更要保持尿管不被压到或扭曲。

I am leaving now, if you have any discomfort, please press the button on the call signal. I will come here as soon as possible. Have a good rest.

我马上要离开了，如果您有什么不适请按呼叫器找我，我会尽快过来帮助您的，好好休息。

Scoring Criteria 11
评分细则 11

项目		总分	技术操作要求	标准分	扣分说明	得分
评估 12	仪表	4	仪表端庄、服装整洁、修剪指甲、洗手、戴口罩	4	一项不符扣2分	
	物品	4	用物齐备，治疗车上下放置合理			
	环境	4	环境符合要求	2	一项不符扣1分	
	患者	4	①病情；②诊断膀胱充盈度；③局部皮肤；④生活自理，能力，如不能自理，协助清洗外阴，合作程度，心理状态；⑤生命体征，意识状态等	4	一项不符扣1分	
实施 68	核对解释	4	核对床号、姓名（处置卡、床头卡）	2	一项不符扣1分	
			解释内容合理（操作目的、配合方法及注意事项）	2	一项不符扣2分	
	初次消毒	18	关闭门窗、遮挡屏风、调节室温（22～24 ℃）	3	一项不符扣1分	
			摆好体位：女性仰卧屈膝位，双下肢屈曲外展，脱下对侧裤子，盖在近侧腿部，对侧腿盖被；男性下肢自然放置略分开	8	一项不符扣2分	
			臀下垫治疗巾方法合理、平整	2	一项不符扣2分	
			检查无菌包正确，放弯盘于外阴处，消毒盘摆放合理	2	一项不符扣1分	
			女性患者：一手戴一次性手套，另一手持镊子，初步消毒阴阜、大阴唇，分开大阴唇，消毒阴唇沟、小阴唇和尿道 男性患者：消毒阴阜、阴茎、阴囊，另一手用无菌纱布裹住阴经，将包皮向后推，暴露尿道口，自尿道口向外向后旋转擦拭尿道口、龟头及冠状沟	3	顺序错误不给分	
	二次消毒	26	检查导尿包方法正确	2	一项不符扣2分	
			打开导尿包方法正确	2	一项不符扣2分	
			无菌面大、平整、双层	2	一项不符扣2分	
			戴手套方法正确	2	一项不符扣2分	
			铺洞巾方法正确，无污染	4	一项不符扣2分	
			放弯盘于洞巾下，无菌区内物品摆放整齐、合理	2	一项不符扣2分	
			取出消毒棉球，放入弯盘内	2	一项不符扣2分	
			检查导尿管及气囊性能，润滑导尿管	4	一项不符扣2分	
			连接集尿袋	1	一项不符扣2分	
			二次消毒外阴方法正确、步骤正确	4	一项不符扣1分	

续表

项目		总分	技术操作要求	标准分	扣分说明	得分
实施 68	插管	10	插管方法正确,见尿后再插入深度合理	4	一项不符扣 2 分	
			向气囊内注水,确定导尿管固定妥当	2	一项不符扣 2 分	
			悬挂尿袋方法正确,位置妥当	2	一项不符扣 2 分	
			摘手套,整理用物	2	一项不符扣 2 分	
	整理	8	整理患者,卧位舒适、床单位整洁	2	一项不符扣 2 分	
			洗手,摘口罩,再核对,健康教育	2	一项不符扣 2 分	
			撤掉屏风、开窗;观察尿液、记录	4	一项不符扣 1 分	
评价 20	熟练	8	动作熟练,步骤合理,掌握相关知识,15 min 内完成职业保护恰当	8	每超过 30 s 扣一分	
	效果	2	患者感觉舒适安全、无不良反应	2	酌情扣分	
	英语	10	发音标准,语言流畅,关爱患者,沟通良好	10	酌情扣分	
主考教师:			日期:	总分:100	得分:	

评分参考:91～100 分为优,81～90 分为良,71～80 分为中,60～70 分为差,低于 60 分为不及格。

Chapter 9 Enema 灌 肠 术

9.1 Large-volume Non-retention Enema 大量不保留灌肠

Purpose 操作目的

1. To relieve constipation and flatulence by softening feces, stimulating peristalsis and initiating the defecation reflex.

通过软化粪便、刺激肠蠕动和引发排便反射来解除便秘和肠胀气。

2. To clean the bowel in preparation for enteric diagnostic examination, surgical or delivery procedure.

清洁灌肠，为肠道诊断性检查、手术或分娩做准备。

3. To detoxify the digestive tract by diluting or removing enteric deleterious material.

通过稀释并清除肠道内的有害物质来减轻中毒。

4. To lower the body temperature for hyperthermia patients by instilling cold solution.

通过灌入低温液体，为高热患者降温。

Assessment 评估

1. Assess the patient's age, level of consciousness, health condition (including

abdominal pain, abdominal distention, bowel movement and mobility status), diagnosis and purpose of large-volume non-retention enema.

评估患者的年龄、意识、病情(包括腹痛、腹胀、排便情况、躯体活动能力等)、诊断及大量不保留灌肠的目的。

2. Assess the patient's ability to control external sphincter of anus.

评估患者肛门括约肌控制能力。

3. Assess the patient's condition of anal skin and mucosa, such as the anal area for soreness, haemorrhoids.

评估患者肛周皮肤、黏膜情况,如有无肛周疼痛、痔疮等。

4. Assess the patient's psychological status, ability to cooperate, communication skills and understanding of large-volume non-retention enema.

评估患者的心理状态、合作程度、表达能力及对大量不保留灌肠的了解程度。

Gather Equipment 物品准备

治疗盘内:disposable enema set 一次性灌肠器(disposable gloves 一次性手套,enema bag 灌肠袋,drape 垫巾),bath thermometer 水温计,swabs 棉签,lubricant 润滑剂。

治疗盘外:treatment sheet 医嘱卡,measuring cup(enema solution as prescribed)量杯(内盛医嘱灌肠液),hand sanitizer 洗手液,kidney basin 弯盘,tissues or toilet paper 卫生纸,bedpan 便盆,medical waste bag 医疗垃圾袋、IV stand/pole 输液架。

Procedure 操作过程

1. Report and tidy your dress.

报告并整理仪表。

2. Check the validity of hand sanitizer and wash hands in 7 steps and put on the mask.

检查洗手液的有效期,7 步洗手法洗手并戴口罩。

3. Gather equipments. Prepare enema solution as prescribed. The type、temperature, concentration and volume of the enema solution should be correct. If preparing 0.1%-0.2% soap solution, fill the measuring cylinder with warm boiled water with appropriate temperature first, then add 10% soap solution. This reduces the amount of suds in the enema solution.

备齐用物。按医嘱准备灌肠液。灌肠液种类、温度、浓度及量都应该正确。如配制0.1% ~ 0.2%肥皂水,可先在量筒内配制合适温度的温开水,再加入10%肥皂水。这样可以减少灌肠液中肥皂液的产生。

4. Wash hands and remove the mask.

洗手,摘口罩。

5. Take the equipment to the ward. Assess the working environment. (The working environment should be at appropriate room temperature and has adequate lighting. Close the doors and windows and provide the privacy environment to the patient by drawing curtains or using screens. Ensure that the toilet is available.)

携用物至病室,评估操作环境。(操作环境应保持合适的室温和充足的光线。关好门窗、拉上窗帘或使用屏风遮挡以保护患者的隐私。确定卫生间随时可用。)

6. Check the patient's bed number and name.

核对床头卡上床号和患者姓名。

7. Take the equipment to the bedside. Check the patient's name. Explain the purpose and procedure of the operation, and get cooperation from the patient.

携用物至患者床旁。核对患者姓名。解释操作目的和过程,取得患者合作。

8. Assess the patient's ability to control external sphincter of anus. Assess the patient's condition of anal skin and mucosa.

评估患者肛门括约肌控制能力及患者肛周皮肤、黏膜情况。

9. Assist the patient to left side-lying position with knees flexed. Remove pants to knees. Move the buttocks to the edge of the bed.

协助患者取左侧卧位,双膝屈膝,裤脱至膝部,臀部移至床沿。

10. For the patient with poor external sphincter control, position him/her in supine position on bedpan.

肛门括约肌控制力差的患者取仰卧位,臀下垫便盆。

11. Cover the patient with a quilt leaving only the buttocks exposed.

盖好盖被,只暴露患者臀部。

12. Check and open the package of a disposable enema set and take out the drape.

检查并打开一次性灌肠器包装,取出治疗巾。

13. Place the drape under the buttocks and a basin near the buttocks. Put toilet paper on the drape.

将垫单铺于臀下,弯盘置于臀边。将卫生纸放于垫巾上。

14. Adjust the height of IV stand/pole from the solution surface to anus to 40-60 cm.

调节输液架高度，使液面距肛门 40～60 cm。

15. Wear disposable gloves.

戴一次性手套。

16. Check the connection of enema bag and tubing.

检查灌肠袋与连接管的连接情况。

17. Close the regulating clamp of the enema tubing.

关闭灌肠袋连接管上的管夹。

18. Add the prepared solution into the enema bag.

将准备好的灌肠液倒入灌肠袋。

19. Hang the enema bag on an IV stand/pole, make the height from the solution surface to anus to 40-60 cm, not more than 30 cm for typhoid patients.

将灌肠袋挂于输液架上，使其液面距肛门 40～60 cm，伤寒患者不得超过 30 cm。

20. Lubricate the tip of the rectal tube.

润滑肛管前端。

21. Release the clamp, and allow the solution to flow enough to fill the tubing for removing air from the tubing, then reclamp the enema tubing.

开放管夹，使溶液充满管道以排尽肛管内气体，然后夹管。

22. With one hand, Separate the buttocks with toilet paper to expose anus.

一手垫着卫生纸分开臀部暴露肛门。

23. Instruct the patient to take deep breaths.

指导患者深呼吸。

24. After you get a good view of the anus, with the other hand, gently insert the tip of rectal tube through the anus into rectum. If it meets obstruction, pull the tube back a little bit and insert it by rotating slowly. The length of insertion varies: 7-10 cm for adults, 4 - 7 cm for children.

看清楚肛门后，另一只手轻轻将肛管经肛门插入直肠。如果插入受阻，则退出少许，边旋转边缓慢插入。插管深度不同：成人 7～10 cm，小儿 4～7 cm。

25. Open the regulating clamp and allow the solution to enter slowly.

开放管夹，使液体缓缓流入。

26. Continue to hold the rectal tube until the end of fluid instillation.

固定肛管直至灌液完毕。

27. Observe the speed of fluid instillation closely. If the solution surface drops too slowly or ceases going, revolve or squeeze the rectal tube gently.

密切观察灌肠袋内液面下降的速度。如液面下降过慢或停止，可轻轻转动或挤捏肛管。

28. Ask the patient to report any discomforts associated with enema administration. If the patient complains of fullness or urges to defecate, ask the patient to take deep breaths, slower the speed of fluid instillation, or make a pause of instillation for a moment in order to relieve the patient's discomforts.

询问患者灌肠中有无不适。如有腹胀或便意,应嘱患者做深呼吸,或减慢灌液流速或暂停灌液片刻,以减轻患者的不适。

29. Observe the patient's response carefully. If tachycardia, facial pallor, diaphoresis, palpitation, short breath or abdominal pain occurs, stop administering enema immediately and notify your doctor.

仔细观察患者的反应。如发现心动过速、面色苍白、出冷汗、心慌、气急或剧烈腹痛时,应立即停止灌肠并及时通知医生。

30. Clamp the enema tubing after all solution is infused or if the patient cannot retain any further solution.

待灌肠液即将流尽或患者实在不能忍受更多灌肠液时夹管。

31. Place layers of toilet paper around the rectal tube at anus and gently remove the tube.

用卫生纸在肛周包裹肛管轻轻拔出。

32. Discard the used enema set into the medical waste bag.

将用过的整套灌肠器放进医疗垃圾袋。

33. Clean the anus, remove gloves.

擦净肛门,脱下手套。

34. Remove the drap and the basin.

撤去治疗巾及弯盘。

35. Assist the patient to put on pants.

协助患者穿好裤子。

36. Explain to the patient that the feeling of distention is normal.

向患者说明有腹胀感是正常现象。

37. Ask the patient to do his/her best to retain solution for 5-10 minutes while lying quietly in bed.

嘱患者安静躺在床上,尽量保留灌肠液 5~10 min 后再排便。

38. Explain to the patient with constipation the importance of maintaining bowel regularity and instruct the preventions of constipation. Not to rely on enemas to maintain bowel regularity because repeated use of enemas will destroy defecation reflex

and lead to further alterations in bowel elimination.

向便秘患者解释维持正常排便习惯的重要性并指导预防便秘的方法。告诉患者不要依赖灌肠，因为长期灌肠会破坏排便反射，引起排便障碍。

39. If enemas are ordered until "clear", warn the patient against flushing the toilet before inspection and report whether the fluid returned is light brown in color with no pieces of stool. If the fluid returned still has stool particles, this enema will be repeated.

如果医嘱为"清洁灌肠"，应提醒患者先观察排出液再冲厕所，并报告排出液是否清亮、无粪渣。如果还有粪渣，需重复灌肠。

40. Post-procedure 整理

(1) Assist the patient to comfortable position. Ask the patient's feelings and needs.

协助患者取舒适体位。询问患者的感受及需求。

(2) Assist the patient to the bathroom or help position on bedpan if necessary. Assist the patient to wash the anal area as needed.

必要时协助患者到洗手间或使用便盆。如有必要，协助患者清洗肛周。

(3) Tidy up the patient's bed.

整理床单位。

(4) Have toilet paper and call signal within patient's reach.

将卫生纸、呼叫器放于患者易取处。

(5) Open the door and windows according to the situation. Remove screens.

酌情开门窗，撤屏风。

(6) Discard all used equipment appropriately.

合理清理用物。

(7) Wash hands and remove the mask.

洗手、摘口罩。

(8) Sign the prescription chart or treatment sheet to indicate that the non-retention enema has been administered.

在医嘱单或治疗单上签名，表示不保留灌肠已执行。

(9) Observe the patient's response to enema, e.g., sweating, weakness and abdominal cramping.

观察患者对灌肠的反应，有无出冷汗、乏力、腹部绞痛等。

(10) Observe the effect of the enema.

观察灌肠的效果。

(11) Document the defecation times after enema on the blank space of the vital sign flowsheet. "2/E" means 2 times of defecation after enema.

在体温单上相应的栏目记录灌肠后的排便次数。"2/E"表示灌肠后解便 2 次。

Nurse Alert 护理事项

1. Enema cannot be administered to pregnancy, patients with acute abdominal pain, GI bleeding or cardiovascular diseases.

妊娠、急腹症、消化道出血及严重心血管疾病等患者禁忌灌肠。

2. For typhoid patients, the volume of enema solution should not be more than 500 mL and the height from the solution surface to anus should not be more than 30 cm.

伤寒患者灌肠时溶液不得超过 500 mL,压力要低(液面不得超过肛门 30 cm)。

3. Soap solution cannot be used for patients with hepatic coma in order to avoid the generation and absorption of ammonia.

为肝昏迷患者灌肠时禁用肥皂水,以减少氨的生成。

4. Accurately control the temperature, concentration, speed of fluid instillation, pressure and volume of the enema solution.

准确掌握灌肠溶液的温度、浓度、流速、压力和溶液的量。

5. Normal saline is not allowed to used for patients with congestive heart failure or with water and sodium retention.

充血性心力衰竭和水钠潴留患者禁用生理盐水灌肠。

6. Incontinent patients should assure supine position on a bedpan because they will not be able to retain all enema solution.

肛门括约肌控制能力差的患者采取平卧位并臀下垫便盆,因为他们无法很好地保留灌肠液。

7. If providing enema for a hyperthermia patient, ask the patient to retain solution for 30 minutes. Take body temperature and document it 30 minutes after defecation.

为高热患者灌肠,嘱患者保留灌肠液 30 min。排便后 30 min 后再测量并记录体温。

New Words and Expressions
单 词 表

enema [ˈenimə] *n.* 灌肠剂(复数 enemas);灌肠治疗
constipation [kɔnstiˈpeiʃən] *n.* [临床] 便秘;受限制
flatulence [ˈflætʃələns] *n.* [内科] 肠胃胀气;浮夸;自负
diagnostic [ˌdaiəgˈnɔstik] *adj.* 诊断的;特征的
external sphincter 外括约肌
haemorrhoids [ˈhemərɔidz] *n.* 痔核;痔疾
typhoid [ˈtaifɔid] *n.* 伤寒
lubricate [ˈluːbrikeit] *vi.* 润滑;涂油;起润滑剂作用 *vt.* 使润滑;给……加润滑油
tachycardia [ˌtækiˈkɑːdiə] *n.* [内科] 心动过速;心跳过速

Communication Model
沟 模 板 通

Self-introduction Model 常规介绍模板

Good morning/afternoon teachers, my name is ××, I come from class ××, my student's number is ××. Today, I am going to show you the process of large-volume non-retention enema, the equipments I have prepared are... ,everything is ready, may I start?

早上/下午好老师,我的名字是××,来自××班,我的学号是××。今天,我要进行的操作是大量不保留灌肠,所准备的用物有……,准备完毕,请求开始。

Assessment 评估

The ward is tidy and well ventilated. There is no patient receiving therapy or dining. The working environment is at appropriate room temperature and has adequate lighting, and can provide the privacy environment to the patient. The toilet is available. The patient is in good mental state, health condition. He/she has the ability to control external sphincter of anus. The condition of anal skin and mucosa is in good condition. The temperature of enema solution is in normal range.

病室整洁、通风良好。没有患者接受治疗或进餐。操作环境室温合适和光线充足。可以保护患者的隐私。卫生间随时可用。患者精神状态、健康状况良好。他/她有能力控制肛门外括约肌。肛周皮肤和黏膜完好。灌肠液的温度在正常范围内。

Communication 沟通

Good morning, sir. I'm your primary nurse, my name is ××. Would you tell me your full name? Is there any abdominal distension or pain? According to the doctor's order, I will provide you with large-volume non-retention enema to relieve constipation and flatulence for you. I will insert a tube through your anus, irrigate quantity of fluid into you rectum. The fluid can soften your feces and stimulate the bowel to eliminate feces easily. Please cooperate with me during the procedure.

早上好,先生。我是您的责任护士,我的名字是××,您能告诉我您的名字吗? 您有没有腹胀或疼痛的感觉? 根据医嘱,我将要为您进行大量不保留灌肠来缓解便秘和肠胀气。我将灌肠管从肛门插入直肠来灌注大量的液体。灌肠液可以软化您的粪便和刺激肠道,使排便更容易。请配合我的操作。

Please lie on left-side position.

请左侧卧位躺好。

Now, I will insert the tube, if you feel uncomfortable, please take a deep mouth breathing.

我将要插管了,如果您觉得不舒服,请张嘴深呼吸。

Are you OK with this position? Please do not go to bathroom immediately, you should keep the fluid for 10 minutes and it will be effective.

您觉得这个位置舒服吗? 请您不要立即去卫生间,您应该保留灌肠液 10 min 才有效。

There is a bedpan on the chair, the call signal is here, if you need any help please press the button on the call signal, I will be there to do you a favour. Have a good rest.

便盆已放在椅子上,呼叫器在这里,如果您需要帮助,请按呼叫器,我将过来帮助您。好好休息。

Scoring Criteria 12
评分细则 12

项目		总分	技术操作要求	标准分	扣分说明	得分
评估 12	仪表	4	仪表端庄、服装整洁、修剪指甲、洗手、戴口罩	4	一项不符扣 2 分	
	物品	4	用物齐备、放置合理，灌肠液配制正确	2	一项不符扣 1 分	
	环境		环境符合要求	2	一项不符扣 2 分	
	患者	4	了解患者诊断、意识状态、合作程度、身体状况	2	一项不符扣 1 分	
			肛周皮肤、黏膜情况	2	一项不符扣 1 分	
实施 66	核对解释	6	核对床号、姓名	2	一项不符扣 1 分	
			解释内容合理(操作目的、配合方法)	4	一项不符扣 2 分	
	灌肠	52	根据患者情况选择合适体位(两种，左、右侧卧位)	2	一项不符扣 2 分	
			体位舒适，方便操作，保暖良好	6	一项不符扣 2 分	
			铺洞巾动作轻柔，弯盘位置放置恰当	4	一项不符扣 1 分	
			灌肠筒高度适宜(40～60 cm)	2	一项不符扣 2 分	
			肛管润滑充分	2	一项不符扣 2 分	
			连接肛管无污染	6	污染一次扣 2 分	
			排气方法正确，溶液不沾湿床单、地面	2	一项不符扣 2 分	
			插管时请患者配合恰当，动作轻，手法正确	4	一项不符扣 2 分	
			肛管插入深度为 7～10 cm	2	一项不符扣 4 分	
			固定肛管不脱出	2	一项不符扣 2 分	
			正确观察液体流入情况、处理正确	2	一项不符扣 2 分	
			及时观察患者情况(两种：①面色、腹痛；②液面、便意)，处理正确(对应处理)	8	一项不符扣 4 分	
			拔管方法正确，止血钳夹闭或关闭开关	4	一项不符扣 2 分	
			用后肛管放置妥当	2	一项不符扣 2 分	
			指导保留时间	2	一项不符扣 2 分	
			正确协助患者排便	2	一项不符扣 2 分	
	整理	8	患者卧位舒适，衣物整洁	2	一项不符扣 2 分	
			床单位整洁	2	一项不符扣 2 分	
			用物处理正确，洗手、记录	4	一项不符扣 2 分	
评价 22	熟练	8	动作轻稳、熟练，步骤合理	2	一项不符扣 2 分	
			相关理论知识掌握熟练	2	一项不符扣 2 分	
			按规定时间完成(10 min)	4	每超过 30 s 扣 1 分	
	效果	4	患者感觉安全舒适，无不良反应	4	酌情扣分	
	英语	10	发音标准，语言流畅，关爱患者，沟通有效	10	酌情扣分	
主考教师：			日期：	总分：100	得分：	

评分参考：91～100 分为优，81～90 分为良，71～80 分为中，60～70 分为差，低于 60 分为不及格。

Chapter 10
Administering Injection
注 射 法

10.1 Intradermal Injection
皮内注射

Purpose 操作目的

An intradermal injection is the administration of a medication into the dermal layer of the skin just beneath the epidermis. It is frequently used for allergy testing, vaccination and the first step of local anesthesia.

皮内注射法是将药液注射于表皮与真皮之间的方法，常用于药物过敏试验、预防接种和局麻的起始步骤。

Assessment 评估

1. Assess the patient's age, level of consciousness, health condition, allergy history, medication using and whether the patient is fasting.

评估患者的年龄、意识、病情、过敏史、用药史及是否空腹。

2. Assess the skin condition of injection sites.

评估注射部位的皮肤情况。

3. Assess the patient's psychological status, ability to cooperate, communication skills and knowledge of allergy testing.

评估患者的心理状态、合作程度、表达能力及过敏试验的知识水平。

Gather Equipment 物品准备

治疗盘内：metal file 砂轮，sterile gauzes 无菌纱布，antiseptic solution 消毒液，sterile swabs 无菌棉签，1 mL syringe 1 mL 注射器，prescription chart 医嘱单，prescribed medication 医嘱药液，sterile saline 无菌生理盐水。first-aid kit for allergy testing containing 0.1% adrenalin hydrochloride 药物过敏试验急救盒(内含 0.1%盐酸肾上腺素)。

治疗盘外：kidney basin 弯盘，hand sanitizer 洗手液，sharps container 锐器盒，oxygen equipment 氧气装置，suction equipment 吸痰装置。

Procedure 操作过程

1. Report and tidy your dress.

报告并整理仪表。

2. Check the validity of hand sanitizer and wash hands in 7 steps and put on the mask.

检查洗手液的有效期，7 步洗手法洗手并戴口罩。

3. Gather equipments and check for the prescription and equipments.

备齐用物，核对医嘱及用品。

4. Wash hands and remove the mask.

洗手，摘口罩。

5. Take the equipments to the ward. Assess the working environment.

携用物至病室内。评估操作环境。

6. Check the patient's bed number and name.

核对床头卡上床号和患者姓名。

7. Take the equipments to the bedside. Check the patient's name. Explain the purpose and procedure of the operation, ask for the history of using medication and history of allergy, and if the patient is fasting. Getting cooperation from the patient.

携用物至患者床旁。核对患者姓名。解释操作目的和过程，询问用药史及过敏史，以及患者是否为空腹。取得患者合作。

8. Open the cap of medical waste and garbage bin, wash hands and put on the mask.

打开污物桶(医用垃圾桶、生活垃圾桶)盖,洗手、戴口罩。

9. Check the solution for skin testing against prescription chart, check the expiration date and quality.

根据医嘱单核对试敏液的名称、有效期及质量。

10. Remove the center part of the aluminum cap of the solution. Clean the surface of rubber seal with antiseptic swabs routinely and allow it to dry.

除去铝盖的中心部位,常规消毒瓶塞,待干。

11. Select a 1 mL syringe. Check the manufacture, expiration date and the integrity of its package. Open the package and remove the needle cap from the syringe.

选择一支 1 mL 注射器,检查其生产日期、有效期及包装的完整性,打开外包装并取下护针帽。

12. Withdraw 0.2 mL solution from the vial with the syringe.

用注射器在密封瓶中抽吸 0.2 mL 溶液。

13. Select an appropriate injection site, usually the ventral lower arm. (Avoid scarring skin, pigmentation and hair heavy skin, etc.)

选择合适的注射部位,常选前臂掌侧下段。(避开瘢痕、色素沉着及汗毛较重的皮肤等。)

14. Clean the injection site with alcohol swabs routinely, apply swabs at the center of site and rotate outward in circular direction for about 5 cm, and allow it to dry.

用酒精消毒注射部位,以注射点为圆心向外旋转,消毒范围直径约 5 cm,待干。

15. Recheck the patient's identification and medication. Make sure that there is no air bubble in the syringe and remove the needle cap.

再次核对患者及药名。确保注射器内无气泡,取下护针帽。

16. Grasp the patient's forearm with your left hand, and pull the skin taut on ventral forearm.

用左手握紧前臂,绷紧掌侧皮肤。

17. Hold the syringe with your right hand, and the needle bevel facing up. Insert the needle bevel into the intradermal tissue layer thoroughly at a 5° angle, and then place the syringe flat.

右手持注射器,针尖斜面向上,与皮肤成 5°角进针,将针尖斜面全部刺入皮肤内后放平注射器。

18. Stabilize the needle hub with the thumb of your left hand. Inject 0.1 mL solution for skin testing slowly to form a small bleb/wheal on the skin.

左手拇指固定针栓，缓慢推注皮试液 0.1 mL，使局部皮肤隆起形成一个皮丘。

19. Withdraw the needle quickly with your right hand. Tell the patient not to press on the site.

右手迅速拔针，嘱患者勿按压针眼。

20. Do not recap the needle. Discard the needle into the sharp container immediately.

勿套回针头帽。立即将针头放进锐器盒中。

21. Recheck the patient's name, bed number and the medication. Remind the patient to stay in the room for 20 minutes after the injection, and notify doctor/nurse immediately if there are any unusual effects.

再次核对患者姓名、床号及药名。提醒患者注射后 20 min 内不可离开病室，如有不适及时通知医生或护士。

22. Stay with the patient for the first 5 minutes after the injection. If the patient has no unusual effects, then leave the patient. Assist the patient to comfortable position and tidy up his/her clothing if necessary. Tidy up the bed.

床边观察 5 min，患者无不适才可离开。协助患者取舒适体位，必要时整理衣服，清洁床单位。

23. Put the first-aid kit on the bedside table until the test result is confirmed negative and the patient has no unusual effects. (If the patient feel unwell such as dizziness, flustered, nausea, inform your doctor immediately.)

将急救盒放在床旁桌上，直至试验结果为阴性或患者无不适。（如患者有不适症状，如表现为头晕、心慌、恶心，立即通知医生。）

24. Cover the medical waste and garbage bin, wash hands and remove the mask.

盖上污物桶（医用垃圾桶、生活垃圾桶）盖，洗手、摘口罩。

25. Wash hands and remove the mask. Record the time of administering allergy testing.

洗手、摘口罩。记录过敏试验的执行时间。

26. Return to read the result of the allergy testing 20 minutes after the intradermal injection is finished, and document the result according to local policy (take notes PCTA(－) or PCTA(＋)). Observe closely and record the patient's response to allergy testing.

皮内注射 20 min 后返回病室判断皮试结果，并按照医院要求记录（记录 PCTA(－)或 PCTA(＋)）。严密观察并记录患者对青霉素过敏试验的反应。

Nurse Alert 护理事项

1. Follow the checking procedure; use aseptic techniques, safety injection techniques and standard precautions strictly.

严格执行查对制度、无菌技术、安全注射和标准预防的操作原则。

2. Prepare well before penicillin allergy testing.

做好青霉素过敏试验前的准备。

(1) Ask the patient whether he/she has a history of penicillin allergy. If the patient was ever allergic to penicillin, this skin testing should not be done and notify your doctor.

询问患者有无青霉素过敏史。如果患者曾对青霉素过敏,则不可做此皮试并通知医生。

(2) The patient can not be fasting. For a NOP patient or a patient in the emergency room, allergy testing should be done during or after intravenous infusion.

患者不宜空腹。进食或急诊患者应在输液中或输液后进行过敏试验。

(3) Prepare medication and equipment for an emergency use.

做好急救的药物及物品准备。

(4) Prepare the solution right before allergy testing.

新鲜配制试敏液。

3. Do not clean the injection site with an iodine swab. If the patient is allergic to alcohol, select other colorless skin disinfector.

忌用碘酊消毒注射部位。如果患者对酒精过敏,可选用其他无色溶液的皮肤消毒剂。

4. Assist patients who are too weak or too anxious to supine position to avoid dizziness.

协助体质虚弱或情绪紧张的患者平卧以防晕针。

5. After the injection, remind the patient not to leave his/her room or scratch the small bleb, and to notify doctor /nurse immediately if there are any unusual effects.

注射后,提醒患者不可离开病室,不可揉搓皮丘,如有不适立刻通知医生/护士。

6. If you are not sure of the test result, preform a control testing by intradermally injecting 0.1 mL NS on the other forearm.

如果对皮试结果有怀疑,应在对侧前臂皮内注射生理盐水 0.1 mL 进行对照试验。

7. Notify the patient and his/her family the result of skin testing. If the test result

is positive, document the result in the outpatient medical record, and advise the patient to avoid penicillin.

告知患者及其家属皮试结果。如果结果为阳性，将结果记录在患者门诊病历上，并告知患者应从此避免使用青霉素。

8. For outpatients, make sure that the patient and his/her family know the symptoms and signs of an allergic reaction to the injection and the necessary immediate action, and provide the emergency phone numbers.

对门诊患者，应确保患者及其家属了解过敏反应的症状、体征及必要的急救措施，并提供急救电话。

New Words and Expressions
单 词 表

intradermal [ˌintrə'dəːməl] *adj.* 皮肤内的

injection [in'dʒekʃən] *n.* 注射

administration [ədmini'streiʃən] *n.* (药的)配给；服法；用法；处理(过程)

dermal ['dəːməl] *adj.* 真皮的；皮肤的

layer ['leiə] *n.* 层

beneath [bi'niːθ] *prep.* 在……之下

epidermis [ˌepi'dəːmis] *n.* 上皮，表皮

allergy ['ælədʒi] *n.* 过敏症

vaccination [ˌvæksi'neiʃən] *n.* 接种疫苗

anesthesia [ˌænis'θiːʒə] *n.* 麻醉

file [fail] *n.* 锉刀

adrenalin [ə'drenəlin] *n.* 肾上腺素

container [kən'teinə] *n.* 容器

bin [bin] *n.* 容器

swabs [swɔbs] *n.* 棉签(swab 的复数)

manufacture [mænju'fæktʃə] *n.* 制造；产品

integrity [in'tegriti] *n.* 完整

withdraw [wið'drɔː] *vt.* 抽吸

ventral ['ventr(ə)l] *adj.* 腹侧的；[解剖]腹部的

identification [aiˌdentifi'keiʃən] *n.* 鉴定，识别；认同；身份证明

forearm ['fɔːrɑːm] *n.* 前臂

taut [tɔːt] *adj.* 拉紧的

bevel [ˈbevəl] *n.* 斜角

tissue [ˈtiʃuː] *n.* 组织

thoroughly [ˈθʌrəli] *adv.* 彻底地,完全地

flat [flæt] *n.* 平面

stabilize [ˈstebəlaiz] *vt.* 使稳固

hub [hʌb] *n.* 中心

thumb [θʌm] *n.* 拇指

bleb [bleb] *n.* (皮肤上的)疱

wheal [hwil] *n.* 水疱

Communication Model
沟通模板

Self-introduction Model　常规介绍模板

Good morning/afternoon teachers, my name is ××, I come from class ××, my student's number is ××. Today, I am going to show you the process of intradermal injection, the equipments I have prepared are ... ,everything is ready, may I start?

老师早上/下午好,我的名字是××,来自××班,我的学号是××。今天,我要展示的操作是皮内注射,所准备的用物有……,准备完毕,请求开始。

Assessment　评估

The patient is 20 years old and he is diagnosed with "acute pneumonia". The body temperature is 39.7 ℃,no dyspnea, the left lower chest showed dullness on percussion with moist rales at the end of inspiration on auscultation. Doctor's order: 0.9%NS 2 mL, penicillin G 800000 units IM bid. I will administer penicillin allergy testing for the patient first.

患者,20 岁,被诊断为急性肺炎。体温:39.7 ℃,无呼吸困难,左下胸部叩诊闻及浊音,听诊闻及湿啰音。医嘱:0.9%盐水 2 mL,青霉素 G 800000 单位,肌内注射,一天 2 次。我将先为患者进行青霉素过敏试验。

Communication 沟通

Hello, I'm your duty nurse, my name is ××. May I have your full name?

您好,我是您的责任护士,我叫××。请问您叫什么名字?

You have got pneumonia. Doctor prescribed you penicillin for intramuscular injection. Before giving you the penicillin, I have to do a skin testing for you to make sure that you are not allergic to it.

因您患了肺炎,医生给您开了青霉素肌内注射。在青霉素用药前我必须先给您做个皮试,确保您对青霉素不过敏。

Have you ever used penicillin before? Are you allergic to it? Are you allergic to any other kind of medication? Is there anybody else that is allergic to penicillin? /Have your family members ever been allergic to penicillin or any other medication? Do you feel dizzy or hungry now?

您以前用过青霉素吗? 对其他药物过敏吗? 家里人有谁对青霉素或其他药物过敏很严重吗? 您现在有没有感到头晕或有饥饿感?

Now, I will prepare the medication for you, please roll up your sleeves, I will select the right place for injection. OK, it is there.

现在我要为您准备药液,请挽起袖子,我要为您选择注射部位。这里吧。

May I have your name again? (Second check)

能再告诉我一下您的名字吗?(二次核对)

Please do not be nervous, take it easy, you will feel a little prick, do not move your arm.

不要紧张,放轻松,只是疼一小下,千万不要移开手臂哦!

OK, it is done, do not scratch or press on the injection site, I will be back to check for the result for you in 20 minutes. Mr ××, right? (Third check) If you have any discomfort, press the call signal to contact me at any time. See you then.

好的,完成了。请不要搔抓或用衣物压迫进针处,20 min 后我来为您检查结果。是××先生吗?(三次核对)在过程中如有任何不适,随时按呼叫器找我,好,一会见。

Hello, I am coming now. Please tell your name again? Are you OK? Now I will check skin testing results together with my colleague.

您好,我来了。请您再把您的名字告诉我一次好吗? 您还好吗? 我现在要与我的同事一起来查看皮试结果。

If there is no itching, rashes, nausea and other discomfort, and the skin test result is negative, you can use this drug. I will notify the doctor and prepare intramuscular injection for you, Please wait for a moment, and have a good rest!

注射部位无痒感、红肿,患者无恶心和其他不适,皮试结果为阴性,您可以使用这种药品。我会把皮试结果通知医生并为您准备肌内注射的药物,稍等,先休息一会吧。

New Words and Expressions
单 词 表

pneumonia [njuːˈməuniə] *n.* 肺炎
dyspnea [disˈpniːə] *n.* [内科] 呼吸困难
dullness [ˈdʌlnis] *n.* 浊音
percussion [pəˈkʌʃən] *n.* [临床] 叩诊
moist [mɔist] *adj.* 潮湿的
rales [rɑːlz] *n.* 啰音;水泡音;肺的诊音(rale 的复数)
inspiration [ˌinspəˈreiʃən] *n.* 吸气
auscultation [ˌɔːskəlˈteiʃən] *n.* [临床] 听诊
penicillin [peniˈsilin] *n.* 青霉素
dizzy [ˈdizi] *adj.* 晕眩的
intramuscular [ˌintrəˈmʌskjuːlə] *adj.* 肌肉的
scratch [skrætʃ] *vi.* 抓

Scoring Criteria 13
评分细则 13

项目		总分	技术操作要求	标准分	扣分说明	得分
评估 12	仪表	4	仪表端庄、服装整洁、修剪指甲、洗手、戴口罩	4	一项不符扣 2 分	
	物品	4	物品齐备，在有效期内	2	一项不符扣 1 分	
	环境		环境清洁、安静，光线充足	2	一项不符扣 1 分	
	患者	4	了解患者病情、意识状态及合作程度、注射部位皮肤	4	一项不符扣 1 分	
实施 68	核对解释	10	适时三查七对，内容全面（药物、患者、床头卡共同核对）	4	一项不符扣 2 分	
			根据病情解释皮内注射的操作目的、过程、配合方法，询问三史情况	6	一项不符扣 2 分	
	抽吸药液	18	核对（药名、剂量、浓度、时间、用法及质量正确）	2	一项不符扣 1 分	
			检查注射器质量（有效期、包装、型号）	2	一项不符扣 1 分	
			消毒密封瓶正确（消毒液为酒精），消、划、消	2	一项不符扣 2 分	
			正确使用注射器，不污染	2	一项不符扣 1 分	
			抽吸药液方法正确，不污染	4	一项不符扣 2 分	
			抽吸剂量准确，大于 0.1 mL，排尽空气，无浪费	4	一项不符扣 2 分	
			再次核对，置于无菌盘内备用（空瓶一并放入）	2	一项不符扣 1 分	
	注射	32	摆体位正确	2	一项不符扣 1 分	
			选择注射部位正确（并口述原因）	4	一项不符扣 2 分	
			排尽空气，无浪费	2	一项不符扣 2 分	
			穿刺方法正确（一手紧绷皮肤，一手持注射器，斜面向上，与皮肤呈 5°），无污染	6	一项不符扣 2 分	
			固定方法正确，固定针栓	2	一项不符扣 2 分	
			推注药量正确（0.1 mL）	2	一项不符扣 2 分	
			皮丘符合要求	2	一项不符扣 1 分	
			拔针方法正确，不可按压	2	一项不符扣 2 分	
			健康教育（进针点的保护，20 min 后检查结果）	4	一项不符扣 2 分	
			口述阳性及阴性体征	6	一项不符扣 3 分	
	整理	8	患者卧位舒适，衣物整洁	2	一项不符扣 1 分	
			床单位整洁	2	一项不符扣 2 分	
			用物处理正确，7 步洗手法洗手，记录	4	一项不符扣 1 分	

续表

<table>
<tr><th colspan="2">项　　目</th><th>总分</th><th>技术操作要求</th><th>标准分</th><th>扣分说明</th><th>得分</th></tr>
<tr><td rowspan="5">评价
20</td><td rowspan="3">熟练</td><td rowspan="3">8</td><td>操作轻稳、熟练、步骤合理</td><td>2</td><td>一项不符扣 2 分</td><td></td></tr>
<tr><td>相关理论知识掌握熟练</td><td>2</td><td>酌情扣分</td><td></td></tr>
<tr><td>按规定时间完成(5 min),职业保护恰当</td><td>4</td><td>每过 30 s 扣 1 分</td><td></td></tr>
<tr><td>效果</td><td>2</td><td>患者感觉安全舒适,无不良反应</td><td>2</td><td>酌情扣分</td><td></td></tr>
<tr><td>英语</td><td>10</td><td>发音标准,语言流畅,符合逻辑,沟通良好</td><td>10</td><td>酌情扣分</td><td></td></tr>
<tr><td colspan="3">主考教师签字:</td><td>日期:</td><td colspan="2">总分:100</td><td>得分:</td></tr>
</table>

评分参考:91～100 分为优,81～90 分为良,71～80 分为中,60～70 分为差,低于 60 分为不及格。

注:1. 使用过期物品,该项考核为"不及格"。

2. 未核对患者或核对错误,该项考核为"不及格"。

3. 污染注射器乳头、针头而未考虑更换者,该项考核为"不及格"。

10.2 Subcutaneous Injection 皮下注射法

Purpose 操作目的

1. To introduce a small amount of medication into subcutaneous tissue, when the medication is not suitable for oral route and its absorption is somewhat slower than with intramuscular injection, such as insulin and heparin.

将小剂量药液注入皮下组织,用于不宜口服且比肌内注射吸收慢的药物,如胰岛素和肝素。

2. Be used for vaccination, preoperative medication and local anesthesia.

用于预防接种、手术前用药及局部麻醉。

Assessment 评估

1. Assess the patient's age, level of consciousness, health condition and medication purpose.

评估患者的年龄、意识、病情及用药目的。

2. Assess the patient's nutritional status and condition of skin and subcutaneous tissue of injection sites.

评估患者的营养状况及注射部位皮肤、皮下组织的情况。

3. Assess the patient's psychological status, ability to cooperate, communication skills and understanding of the medication plan.

评估患者的心理状态、合作程度、表达能力及给药计划的了解程度。

Gather equipment 物品准备

治疗盘内：metal file 砂轮，sterile gauzes 无菌纱布，antiseptic solution 消毒液，sterile swabs 无菌棉签，1-2 mL syringe 1～2 mL 注射器，prescribed medication 医嘱用药，sterile saline 无菌生理盐水。

治疗盘外：prescription chart 医嘱单，kidney basin 弯盘，hand sanitizer 洗手液，sharp container 锐器盒。

Procedure 操作过程

1. Report and tidy your dress.

报告并整理仪表。

2. Check the validity of hand sanitizer and wash hands in 7 steps and put on the mask.

检查洗手液的有效期，7 步洗手法洗手并戴口罩。

3. Gather equipments and check for the prescription and equipments.

备齐用物，核对医嘱及用品。

4. Wash hands and remove the mask.

洗手、摘口罩。

5. Take the equipments to the ward. Assess the working environment.

携用物至病室内。评估操作环境。

6. Check the patient's bed number and name.

核对床头卡上床号和患者姓名。

7. Take the equipments to the bedside. Check the patient's name. Explain the purpose and procedure of the operation. Getting cooperation from the patient.

携用物至患者床旁。核对患者姓名。解释操作目的和过程。取得患者合作。

8. Open the cap of medical waste and garbage bin, wash hands and put on the mask.

打开污物桶(医用垃圾桶、生活垃圾桶)盖，洗手、戴口罩。

9. Check the medication label against prescription chart, check the expiration date

and quality.

根据医嘱单核对药物的名称、有效期及质量。

10. Select a 2 mL syringe. Check the manufacture and expiration date, and the integrity of its package. Open the package and remove the needle cap from the syringe.

选择一支 2 mL 注射器，检查其生产日期、有效期及包装的完整性，打开外包装并取下护针帽。

11. Withdraw the correct dosage of medication from an ampule or vial.

从安瓿或密封瓶中抽吸准确剂量药液。

12. Recheck the medication label and dosage against the prescription chart, place the syringe with prepared medication in the tray which is prepared with a sterile drape.

再次核对医嘱单，检查药名、剂量无误后，将备好药液的注射器置于治疗盘无菌治疗巾上。

13. Select an appropriate injection site. Remember to alternate sites each time when injection is given.

选择适当的注射部位。记住每次注射应交替更换注射部位。

14. Assist the patient to comfortable position depending on the site selected and instruct the patient to relax.

根据所选择的注射部位，协助患者采取舒适的体位并指导患者放松。

(1) Upper arms(the lower edge of deltoid): the patient sitting or standing.

上臂(三角肌下缘)：患者取坐位或站位。

(2) Two sides of the abdomen: the patient sitting or supine.

两侧腹壁：患者取坐位或仰卧位。

(3) Anterior thighs: the patient sitting in bed or chair.

大腿前侧：患者坐在床上或椅子上。

15. Clean the injection site with alcohol swabs routinely, apply swabs at the center of site and rotate outward in circular direction for about 5 cm, and allow it to dry.

用酒精消毒注射部位，以注射点为圆心向外旋转，消毒范围约直径 5 cm，待干。

16. Recheck the patient's identification and medication. Make sure that there is no air bubble in the syringe and remove the needle cap.

再次核对患者及药名。确保注射器内无气泡，取下护针帽。

17. Hold the skin taut with one hand. With the other hand, hold the syringe with the needle bevel facing up, insert 1/2 to 2/3 of the needle shaft quickly into the subcutaneous tissue at a 30°-40° angle, and stabilize the hub of the needle(If the site

selected is on the abdominal wall, pinch up the skin at least two fingerbreadths from umbilicus to avoid umbilical veins, and insert the needle at a 90° angle).

一手绷紧皮肤，另一只手持注射器，针尖斜面向上，与皮肤成 30°～40°角，快速刺入皮下，深度为针梗的 1/2～2/3，固定针栓（如果选择腹壁注射，应捏起皮肤，距离脐窝至少两横指宽以避开脐静脉，以 90°角进针）。

18. Slowly pull back on plunger to aspirate medication. If no blood appears inject the solution slowly, and observe the patient's response.

慢慢抽动活塞。若无回血则缓慢推注药液，并观察患者的反应。

19. After the injection, withdraw the needle quickly and press on the site with a dry swab until any bleeding stops.

注射完毕，快速拔针并用干棉签按压针刺处至不出血为止。

20. Do not recap the needle. Discard the needle into the sharp container immediately.

勿套回针头帽。分离注射器及针头，将针头立即放进锐器盒中。

21. Recheck the patient's name, bed number and the medication.

再次核对患者姓名、床号及药名。

22. Remind the patient to eat 30 minutes after insulin injection.

提醒患者注射胰岛素后 30 min 再进食。

23. Ask the patient to notify doctor/nurse immediately if there are any unusual effects.

告知患者如有不适，应立即通知医生或护士。

24. Assist the patient to comfortable position and tidy up his/her clothing if necessary. Tidy up the bed. Discard all used equipments appropriately.

帮助患者取舒适卧位，必要时整理衣服，清洁床单位，合理清理用物。

25. Cover the medical waste and garbage bin, wash hands and remove the mask.

盖上污物桶（医用垃圾桶、生活垃圾桶）盖。洗手，摘口罩。

26. Record the medication name, dosage, route and time of administration, and the patient's response.

记录药物名称、剂量、给药途径、给药时间及患者的反应。

Nurse Alert 护理事项

1. Follow the checking procedure; use aseptic techniques, safety injection

techniques and standard precautions strictly.

严格执行查对制度、无菌技术、安全注射和标准预防的操作原则。

2. Select an appropriate injection site. Avoid areas of hardness, inflammation, lesions or scars.

选择合适的注射部位,避免在有硬结、炎症、皮肤受损或瘢痕处进针。

3. If the patient must receive frequent subcutaneous injections, injection sites need to be alternated in an orderly fashion. If necessary, instruct the patient to massage or use warm compress on the site after the injections to prevent tissue fibrosis. But these methods are contraindicated for insulin injections because they can cause faster adsorption. They are also contraindicated for heparin injections because they can cause subcutaneous bleeding.

如果患者需长期皮下注射,应有计划地更换注射部位。必要时,指导患者注射后局部按摩或热敷,以防局部产生硬结。但胰岛素注射后禁用这些方法,以免提早产生吸收。肝素注射后也禁用这些方法,以免出现皮下出血。

4. Select appropriate depth and site to insert according to the patient's nutritional status. Do not insert medications into muscle. For thinner patients, pinch up the skin and insert the needle at an angle of not more than 45°. For special medications such as low-molecular-weight Heparin Calcium injection, pick up the skin and insert the needle at a 90° angle on the abdominal wall.

根据患者的营养状况选择适当的进针深度及部位,不可将药液注入肌肉。对过于消瘦的患者,护士可捏起局部皮肤,进针角度不宜超过 45°;对于特殊药物如低相对分子质量肝素钙注射液,应在腹壁捏起局部皮肤,以 90°角进针注射。

5. Prepare food for patients before insulin injection and remind patients to eat 30 minutes after administering injection(or follow medication directions).

注射胰岛素前应准备好食物,并提醒患者注射后 30 min 进食(或按药品说明书的要求)。

6. After the injection, avoid recapping the needle. Discard the needle-syringe unit into the sharp container immediately to avoid needlestick injuries and contamination. Make sure the injection site has no bleeding before you leave the patient.

注射完毕,避免套回针头帽。不分离针头与注射器,整套立即放进锐器盒,以防针刺伤及被污染。离开患者时,应确保注射部位无出血。

7. The insulin-dependent patients may have to learn how to self-administer injections. It is necessary to teach patients the aseptic principles, basic pharmacology of

insulin, selection of sites and alternating injection sites and injection techniques.

胰岛素依赖型患者应学会自我注射，有必要教会他们无菌技术的操作原则、胰岛素的基本药理知识、注射部位的选择、更换注射部位的方法及注射技术。

New Words and Expressions
单 词 表

subcutaneous [ˌsʌbkjuːˈteiniəs] *adj.* 皮下的；皮下用的
absorption [əbˈsɔːpʃən] *n.* 吸收；全神贯注，专心致志
insulin [ˈinsjulin] *n.* 胰岛素
heparin [ˈhepərin] *n.* [生化] 肝素(用于防治血栓形成等)；肝磷脂
preoperative [priːˈɔpərətiv] *adj.* 外科手术前的；操作前的
ampule [ˈæmpjuːl] *n.* [药] 安瓿
vial [ˈvaiəl] *n.* 小瓶；药水瓶
deltoid [ˈdeltɔid] *n.* 三角肌
abdomen [ˈæbdəmən] *n.* 腹部；下腹；腹腔
anterior [ænˈtiəriə] *adj.* 前面的；先前的
routinely [ruːˈtiːnli] *adv.* 例行公事地；常规地
rotate [ˈrəuteit] *vi.* 旋转；循环
fingerbreadths [ˈfiŋgəbreθ] *n.* 指宽；指幅(为 3/4 英寸到 1 英寸宽)
umbilicus [ʌmˈbilikəs] *n.* 脐，种脐；中心
vein [ven] *n.* 静脉；纹理
plunger [ˈplʌndʒə] *n.* [机] 活塞；潜水者；跳水者；莽撞的人
aspirate [ˈæspəreit] *n.* 送气音；抽出物
recap [ˈriːkæp] *vt.* 不套，不盖

Communication Model
沟 通 模 板

Self-introduction Model 常规介绍模板

Good morning/afternoon teachers, my name is ××, I come from class ××, my student's number is ××. Today, I am going to show you the process of hypodermic injection, the equipments I have prepared are..., everything is ready, may I start?

老师早上/下午好，我的名字是××，来自××班，我的学号是××。今天，我要展示的操作是皮下注射，所准备的用物有……，一切准备完毕，请求开始。

Assessment 评估

Bed 5, Helen Nima, female, 55 years old, business woman. She was admitted due to "Type 2 Diabetes". The doctor's order: Novolin-R 8 units H tid 30 minutes before a meal. The patient is in good mental state and has the ability to cooperate with me.

5号床，海伦尼玛，女，55岁，女商人。她被确诊为"2型糖尿病"。医嘱：餐前30 min，皮下注射，胰岛素诺和灵R 8单位。患者精神状态良好，可以配合皮下注射。

Communication 沟通

Good morning, sir. I'm your duty nurse, you can call me ××. May I have your full name please? OK, In order to control your blood glucose level, I will inject insulin in your subcutaneous tissue routinely as the doctor's order. Do you feel dizzy now?

早上好，我是您的责任护士，我叫××。请问您叫什么名字？为了给您控制血糖水平，遵医嘱今天还是常规皮下注射胰岛素。您现在感觉晕眩吗？

OK, please roll up your sleeve and show your upper arm. I am going to select the right site and clean the skin, you will feel a little cold.

请将衣袖挽起来让我查看下您的上臂，我要为您选择合适的注射部位并消毒皮肤，您可能会觉得有些凉。

Would you like tell me your name again? (Second check)

您能告诉我您的名字吗？(二次核对)

OK, now, I will insert the needle. You will feel a little prick, but don't be nervous, take it easy, breath deeply and do not move your arm.

我现在为您注射。您会感到一点点疼，请不要紧张，放轻松，深呼吸，千万不要移开手臂哦！

OK, it is done. Mr ××, right? (Third check) Don't forget to have your lunch 30 minutes later. If you are not feeling well such as feeling dizzy or sweating, please press the button on the call signal. I will come here to help you. Have a good rest. See you then.

完成了，是××先生吗？（三次核对）不要忘记在注射后 30 min 进餐。如果您感觉晕眩或出冷汗，请立即按呼叫器找我，我会马上过来帮助您。好好休息，一会见。

New Words and Expressions
单 词 表

glucose [ˈgluːkəus] *n.* 葡萄糖

sleeve [sliːv] *n.* 套筒、袖子

sweating [ˈswetiŋ] *n.* 发汗

Scoring Criteria 14
评分细则 14

项目		总分	技术操作要求	标准分	扣分说明	得分
评估 12	仪表	4	仪表端庄、服装整洁、修剪指甲、洗手、戴口罩	4	一项不符扣 2 分	
	物品	4	物品齐备，在有效期内	2	一项不符扣 1 分	
	环境		环境清洁、安静，光线充足，必要时用屏风遮挡	2	一项不符扣 1 分	
	患者	4	了解患者病情、意识状态及合作程度、注射部位皮肤情况	4	一项不符扣 1 分	
实施 66	核对解释	8	核对（床号、姓名；处置卡、床头卡共同核对）	6	每次查对不符各扣 2 分	
			根据病情解释皮下注射的操作目的、过程、配合方法	2	一项不符扣 1 分	
	抽吸药液	20	核对（药名、剂量、浓度、时间、用法及质量正确）	2	一项不符扣 1 分	
			检查注射器质量	2	一项不符扣 1 分	
			消毒密封瓶正确	2	一项不符扣 2 分	
			正确使用注射器，不污染	4	一项不符扣 2 分	
			抽吸药液方法正确，不污染	4	一项不符扣 2 分	
			抽吸剂量准确，排尽空气，无浪费	4	一项不符扣 2 分	
			再次核对，置于无菌盘内备用	2	一项不符扣 1 分	
	注射	30	摆体位正确	2	一项不符扣 2 分	
			选择注射部位正确（并口述正确）	2	一项不符扣 2 分	
			消毒方法、范围（5 cm×5 cm）正确	2	一项不符扣 2 分	
			二次排气，无浪费	4	一项不符扣 2 分	
			穿刺方法正确（进针角度：与穿刺皮肤成 30°～40°，深度正确），无污染	8	一项不符扣 2 分	
			固定方法正确，抽回血正确	4	一项不符扣 2 分	
			推注药物方法正确（缓慢推注，观察患者反应）	2	一项不符扣 1 分	
			拔针方法正确	2	一项不符扣 1 分	
			按压正确	2	一项不符扣 2 分	
			健康教育	2	一项不符扣 1 分	
	整理	8	患者卧位舒适，衣物整洁	2	一项不符扣 1 分	
			床单位整洁	2	一项不符扣 2 分	
			用物处理正确，7 步洗手法洗手，记录	4	一项不符扣 1 分	

续表

项目		总分	技术操作要求	标准分	扣分说明	得分
评价 22	熟练	10	操作轻稳、熟练，理论知识扎实	2	一项不符扣 2 分	
			无菌观念强	4	酌情扣分	
			按规定时间完成(5 min)，职业保护恰当	4	每超过 30 s 扣 1 分	
	效果	2	患者感觉安全舒适，无不良反应	2	酌情扣分	
	沟通	10	发音标准，语言流畅，关爱患者，沟通良好	10	酌情扣分	
主考教师签字：			日期：	总分：100	得分：	

评分参考：91～100 分为优，81～90 分为良，71～80 分为中，60～70 分为差，低于 60 分为不及格。

注：1. 使用过期物品，该项考核为“不及格”。

2. 未核对患者或核对错误，该项考核为“不及格”。

3. 污染注射器乳头、针头而未考虑更换者，该项考核为“不及格”。

4. 未戴口罩者，该项考核为“不及格”。

10.3 Intramuscular Injection 肌内注射法

Purpose 操作目的

To introduce medication into muscle when the medication is not suitable for oral or intravenous route and when more rapid absorption than subcutaneous injection is desired.

将药液注入肌肉，用于不宜口服或静脉注射的药物，且要求比皮下注射发挥更快药效时。

Assessment 评估

1. Assess the patient's age, level of consciousness, health condition and medication purpose.

评估患者的年龄、意识、病情及用药目的。

2. Assess the patient's nutritional status and condition of skin, subcutaneous tissue and muscle of injection sites.

评估患者的营养状况及注射部位皮肤、皮下组织、肌肉组织的情况。

3. Assess the patient's psychological status, ability to cooperate, communication

skills and understanding of the medication plan.

评估患者的心理状态、合作程度、表达能力及对给药计划的了解程度。

Gather equipment 物品准备

治疗盘内：metal file 砂轮，sterile gauzes 无菌纱布，antiseptic solution 消毒液，sterile swabs 无菌棉签，2-5 mL syringe 2-5 mL 注射器，prescribed medication 医嘱用药，sterile saline 无菌生理盐水。

治疗盘外：prescription chart 医嘱单，kidney basin 弯盘，hand sanitizer 洗手液，sharp container 锐器盒。

Procedure 操作过程

1. Report and tidy your dress.

报告并整理仪表。

2. Check the validity of hand sanitizer and wash hands in 7 steps and put on the mask.

检查洗手液的有效期，用7步洗手法洗手并戴口罩。

3. Gather equipments and check for the prescription and equipments.

备齐用物，核对医嘱及用品。

4. Wash hands and remove the mask.

洗手，摘口罩。

5. Take the equipment to the ward. Assess the working environment.

携用物至病室内。评估操作环境。

6. Check the patient's bed number and name.

核对床头卡上床号和患者姓名。

7. Take the equipment to the bedside. Check the patient's name. Explain the purpose and procedure of the operation. Getting cooperation from the patient.

携用物至患者床旁。核对患者姓名。解释操作目的和过程。取得患者合作。

8. Open the cap of medical waste and garbage bin, wash hands and put on the mask.

打开污物桶（医用垃圾桶、生活垃圾桶）盖，洗手、戴口罩。

9. Check the medication against prescription chart, check the expiration date and quality.

根据医嘱单核对药物的名称、有效期及质量。

10. Select a 5 mL syringe. Check the manufacture and expiration date, and the integrity of its package. Open the package and remove the needle cap from the syringe.

选择一只 5 mL 注射器，检查其生产日期、有效期及包装的完整性，打开外包装并取下护针帽。

11. Withdraw the correct dosage of medication from an ampule or vial. Excreting excess gas.

从安瓿或密封瓶中抽吸准确药液。排出多余气体。

12. (Second check) Recheck the medication label and dosage against the prescription chart, place the syringe with prepared medication in the tray which is prepared with a sterile drape. Prepare one dry swab.

(二次核对)再次核对医嘱单，检查药名、剂量无误后，将备好药液的注射器置于治疗盘无菌治疗巾上。拿取干棉签。

13. Explain to patient the effect and side effects of the medication, and pain relieving techniques and precautions.

告知患者药物的作用及副作用、减轻疼痛的配合技巧及注意事项。

14. Select an appropriate injection site. Remember to alternate sites each time injection are given. Assist the patient to comfortable position depending on the site selected: sitting, lying on the side, back or abdomen. Instruct the patient to relax the muscle.

选择适当的注射部位。记住每次注射改变部位。根据注射部位协助患者采取舒适体位:坐位、侧卧位、仰卧位或俯卧位。指导患者放松肌肉。

15. Locate the site using anatomic landmarks.

运用体表解剖标志法定位。

(1) Drawing a cross: Draw an imaginary horizontal line from the top of the gluteal cleft to the left or right lateral aspect of the buttock. Draw an imaginary vertical line down the crest of the ilium, divide the buttock into four quadrants. Inject in the upper outer quadrant of the buttock.

十字法:从臀裂顶点向左或右划一水平线，从髂嵴最高点作一垂线，将一侧臀部划分为四个象限，其外上象限为注射部位。

(2) Drawing a line: Draw an imaginary line from the anterior superior iliac spine to the end of coccyx, divide this line into three equal parts. The upper outer 1/3 is the area for an injection.

连线法:从髂前上棘至尾骨作一连线，其外上 1/3 处为注射部位。

(3) Locating the ventrogluteal site for an intramuscular injection: The tips of the nurse's index and middle fingers are placed respectively on the anterior superior iliac spine and the lower edge of the iliac crest. The triangle formed by the crest of the ilium. The index finger and the middle finger is the injection site.

臀中肌、臀小肌注射定位法：以食指指尖和中指指尖分别置于髂前上棘和髂嵴下缘处，髂嵴、食指、中指之间构成的三角形区域为注射部位。

(4) Locating the vastus lateralis site for an intramuscular injection: The middle third of the muscle on the anterior lateral aspect of the thigh is the injection site.

股外侧肌定位法：大腿中段外侧为注射区。

(5) Locating the deltoid site for an intramuscular injection: The deltoid muscle is found on the lateral aspect of the upper arm. The injection site is 2-3 finger breadths below the acromion process. The deltoid muscle may be used for a small-volume injection.

三角肌定位法：上臂外侧，肩峰下 2～3 横指处为注射部位。可用于小剂量注射。

16. Clean the injection site with antiseptic swabs routinely, apply a swab at the center of site and rotate outward in circular direction for about 5 cm, and allow it to dry.

常规消毒注射部位，以注射点为圆心向外旋转，消毒范围约直径 5 cm，待干。

17. Recheck the patient's identification and medication. Make sure there is no air bubble in the syringes and remove the needle cap.

再次核对患者及药名，确保注射器内无气泡，取下护针帽。

18. Hold the skin taut with one hand. Hold the syringe with the other hand and insert the needle quickly into the muscle at a 90°angle and stabilize the hub of the needle.

一手绷紧皮肤，另一手持注射器以 90°角将针头快速刺入肌内，并固定针栓。

19. Slowly pull back on plunger. If no blood appears, inject the solution slowly and observe the patient's response to medication.

缓慢抽动活塞。若无回血则慢慢推注药液，并观察患者的反应。

20. After the injection, withdraw the needle quickly and press on the site with a dry swab until any bleeding stops.

注射完毕，快速拔针并用干棉签按压针刺处至不出血为止。

21. Do not recap the needle. Discard the needle into the sharp container immediately.

勿套回针头帽。分离注射器及针头，将针头立即放进锐器盒中。

22. (Third check) Recheck the patient's name, bed number and the medication.

(三次核对)再次核对患者姓名、床号及药名。

23. Ask the patient to notify doctor/nurse immediately if there are any unusual effects.

告知患者如有不适,应立即通知医生或护士。

24. Instruct the patient how to use call signal and have it within patient's reach.

指导患者呼叫器的使用方法,并将其放于患者易取处。

25. Cover the medical waste and garbage bin, wash hands and remove the mask. Record the time of administering.

盖上污物桶(医用垃圾桶、生活垃圾桶)盖。洗手、摘口罩。记录执行时间。

Nurse Alert 护理事项

1. Follow the checking procedure, use aseptic techniques, safety injection techniques and standard precautions strictly.

严格执行查对制度、无菌技术、安全注射和标准预防的操作原则。

2. Select an appropriate injection site. Avoid areas of hardness, infection, lesions or scars.

选择合适的注射部位,避免在有硬结、炎症、皮肤受损或瘢痕处进针。

3. Select correct injection site to avoid injuring underlying nerves, bones or blood vessels, especially the sciatic nerve.

选择正确的注射部位,以避免损伤神经、骨骼及血管,尤其是坐骨神经。

4. The dorsogluteal muscle should not be used for children under 2 years old, because the muscle is not fully developed. The ventrogluteal is the preferred injection site for children in order to prevent the injury of sciatic nerve.

对于2岁以下婴儿不宜选用臀大肌注射,因其臀大肌尚未发育好。最好选用臀中肌、臀小肌注射,以免损伤坐骨神经。

5. If the patient must receive frequent intramuscular injections, injection sites need to be alternated and longer needles should be selected. Instruct the patient to massage or use warm compress on the site after the injections to prevent tissue fibrosis.

如果患者需要长期肌内注射,应交替更换注射部位并选用细长的针头。指导患者注射后局部按摩或热敷,以防产生局部硬结。

6. Don't insert the needle all the way in, because it is difficult to remove a needle

if it breaks. If a needle breaks during injection, reassure your patient, ask him/her not to move, stabilize the site, and try to remove the broken needle using sterile hemostat forceps. If the broken needle is hard to retrieve, surgical removal may be required.

进针时,切勿将针头全部刺入,以防断针难以取出。一旦注射时发生断针,先稳定患者情绪,并嘱咐患者原地不动,固定局部组织,尽快用无菌止血钳夹住断端后取出。如断端难以找到,应速请外科医生处理。

7. If blood appears in the syringe on aspiration after inserting the needle, it means the needle is in a blood vessel. If this occurs, stop the injection, withdraw the needle and replace with a new one, and inject at another site. Do not inject the medication into a blood vessel.

进针后如果回抽发现注射器内有回血,说明针头刺入了血管。一旦发生这种情况,应停止注射,拔出针头并更换新针头,另选部位重新注射。不可将药液注射入血管内。

8. Use special techniques to minimize the pain during injections: ① assist the patient to comfortable position and encourage him/her to relax the muscle you will be injecting; ②distract the patient by talking to the patient during injections; ③ if the medication is irritating, change the needle deeper after drawing up the medication; ④prevent antiseptic from clinging to needle during insertion by waiting until the skin is dry; ⑤reduce puncture pain by "darting" the needle; ⑥ or use Z-track technique; ⑦ inject medication slowly and steadily, hold the syringe steadily; ⑧withdraw the needle quickly after injection.

应采用减轻患者疼痛的注射技术:①协助患者协助患者取舒适体位,鼓励患者放松局部肌肉;②注射中与患者沟通,分散其注意力;③如果药物刺激性较强,抽吸药液后更换新的细长针头注射,且进针要深;④需等消毒皮肤的消毒液干后才进针,防止消毒液随针头进入组织;⑤采用快速进针法(飞针法);⑥或采用 Z 型注射技术;⑦缓慢、均匀推注药液并稳固注射器;⑧注射完毕快速拔针。

9. If the patient needs more than one medication injecting at the same time, make sure that no medication incompatibilities exist.

如果患者需同时注射多种药物,应确保药物没有配伍禁忌。

10. After the injection, avoid recapping the needle. Discard the needle-syringe unit into the sharp container immediately to avoid needlestick injuries and contamination. Make sure the injection site has no bleeding before you leave the patient.

注射完毕,避免套回针头帽。不分离针头与注射器,整套立即放进锐器盒,以防针刺伤及被污染。离开患者时,应确保注射部位无出血。

New Words and Expressions
单 词 表

oral [ˈɔːrəl] *adj.* 口腔的，口头的

intravenous [ˌintrəˈviːnəs] *adj.* 静脉内的

alternate [ɔːlˈtəːneit] *n.* 替换物

anatomic [ˌænəˈtɔmik] *adj.* 组织的；解剖学上的；结构上的

landmark [ˈlændmɑːk] *n.* 地标，陆标；标志

imaginary [iˈmædʒinəri] *adj.* 虚构的，假想的；想象的；虚数的

horizontal [ˌhɔriˈzɔntəl] *n.* 水平线，水平面；水平位置

gluteal [ˈgluːtiəl] *adj.* 臀肌的；近臀肌的

lateral [ˈlætərəl] *adj.* 侧面的，横向的

buttock [ˈbʌtək] *n.* 臀部

vertical [ˈvəːtikəl] *n.* 垂直线，垂直面

crest [krest] *n.* [物] 波峰；冠；山顶；顶饰

ilium [ˈiliəm] *n.* [解剖]髂骨；[解剖]肠骨

quadrants [ˈkwɔdrənts] *n.* 象限(quadrant 的复数)

upper [ˈʌpə] *adj.* 上面的，上部的；较高的

superior [suːˈpiəriə] *n.* 上级，长官；优胜者，高手；长者

iliac [ˈiliæk] *adj.* 髂骨的；肠骨的；回肠的

coccyx [ˈkɔksiks] *n.* 尾骨；尾椎

triangle [ˈtraiæŋgl] *n.* 三角(形)

vastus [ˈvæstəs] *n.* 股肌

lateralis [ˈlætərəlis] *n.* 侧体

breadths [breθ] *n.* 宽度，幅度；宽宏

acromion [əˈkrəumjən] *n.* [解剖]肩峰

Communication Model
沟 通 模 板

Self-introduction Model 常规介绍模板

Good morning/afternoon teachers, my name is ××, I come from class ××, my student' s number is ××. Today, I am going to show you the process of intramuscular injection, the equipments I have prepared are..., everything is ready, may I start?

早上/下午好老师,我的名字是××,来自××班,我的学号是××。今天,我要展示的操作是肌内注射,所准备的用物有……,准备完毕,请求开始。

Assessment 评估

Bed 4, Robert Walker, male, 20 years old, college student. Penicillin allergy testing was done and the result was negative.

4号床,罗伯特·沃克,男,20岁,大学生。青霉素试敏结果阴性。

Communication 沟通

Good morning, sir. I'm your duty nurse, you can call me ××. May I have your full name please? OK, Mr ××, The doctor said that your absorption impediment causes the lack of vitamin B_{12}. Hence, he advises you to get injected. Your symptoms will alleviated after a while. You look scare about the injection. Don't be nerves. I will try my best to ease your pain. OK, to ensure your privacy, let me close the curtain.

早上好,我是您的责任护士,您可以叫我××,能告诉我您的名字吗? ××先生,医生说您吸收障碍导致维生素 B_{12} 缺乏,遵医嘱给您注射维生素 B_{12}。一段时间内您的症状就会改善的,您看上去对注射有些害怕。我会用最好的操作减轻您的疼痛,请您不要紧张,为了保证您的隐私,我为您拉上围帘。

Selecting the site 选部位

Which side of your hip do you prefer to get the injection?

您哪侧注射方便呢？

Shall I have a look at your injection site?

让我看看您的注射部位好吗？

It is neither red and swollen or clumpy. Just for a moment, I will give you a shot. Do you have hypersensitive test or any other surgeries? I need to prepare the equipments first, you can go to the washroom. See you then.

您的注射部位没有红肿、硬结。一会儿我就在这给您注射，您现在还有试敏和其他治疗吗？您现在可以去卫生间，我回去准备一下物品，我们一会见。

Second check 二次核对

Could you say your name again?

再告诉我您的名字好吗？

Now I'm going to give you the injection. Have you gone to the bathroom? Which position do you prefer, sit or lie on the side? Please bend your knee slightly, extend your thigh. Do you feel comfortable with this?

现在我要给您做肌内注射了。您去卫生间了吗？您取坐位还是侧卧位呢？请您下腿稍弯曲，上腿伸直，这样您舒服吗？

Pull the trigger 推药

Do you feel pain? There might be a kind of swelling. If any uncomforting reaction occurs, tell me immediately.

您现在感觉痛吗？注射时可能会有些肿胀，如有不适请告诉我。

Third check 三次核对

Hello, may I have your name? OK, I have finished your injection. Thank you for your cooperation. Is there anything else you need? You'd better have a good rest as well as stick to treatment. Call me, if necessary, I will come to see you at any time.

您好，能告诉我您的名字吗？好的，肌内注射已经完成了，谢谢您的配合。您还有什么需要吗？那好，您好好休息，坚持治疗。有事您随时叫我，我也会随时来看您的。

New Words and Expressions
单 词 表

privacy ['praivəsi] *n.* 隐私；秘密；隐居；隐居处

curtain ['kə:tən] *n.* 幕；窗帘

hip [hip] *n.* 臀部

Scoring Criteria 15
评分细则 15

<table>
<tr><th colspan="2">项　目</th><th>总分</th><th>技术操作要求</th><th>标准分</th><th>扣分说明</th><th>得分</th></tr>
<tr><td rowspan="4">评估
12</td><td>仪表</td><td>4</td><td>仪表端庄、服装整洁、修剪指甲、洗手、戴口罩</td><td>4</td><td>一项不符扣 2 分</td><td></td></tr>
<tr><td>物品</td><td rowspan="2">4</td><td>用物备齐，治疗车上、下放置合理</td><td>2</td><td>一项不符扣 1 分</td><td></td></tr>
<tr><td>环境</td><td>环境清洁、安静，光线充足，必要时用屏风遮挡</td><td>2</td><td>一项不符扣 1 分</td><td></td></tr>
<tr><td>患者</td><td>4</td><td>了解患者病情、意识状态及合作程度、注射部位皮肤情况、用药史、过敏史、家族史</td><td>4</td><td>一项不符扣 1 分</td><td></td></tr>
<tr><td rowspan="24">实施
62</td><td rowspan="2">核对
解释</td><td rowspan="2">12</td><td>适时三查七对，内容全面（药物、患者、床头卡共同核对）</td><td>9</td><td>每次查对
不符各扣 3 分</td><td></td></tr>
<tr><td>根据病情解释肌内注射的操作目的、过程、配合方法</td><td>3</td><td>一项不符扣 1 分</td><td></td></tr>
<tr><td rowspan="7">抽吸
药液</td><td rowspan="7">20</td><td>核对（药名、剂量、浓度、时间、用法及质量正确）</td><td>2</td><td>一项不符扣 1 分</td><td></td></tr>
<tr><td>检查注射器质量</td><td>2</td><td>一项不符扣 1 分</td><td></td></tr>
<tr><td>消毒安瓿方法正确（弹—划痕—消毒—折断）</td><td>2</td><td>一项不符扣 2 分</td><td></td></tr>
<tr><td>正确使用注射器，不污染</td><td>4</td><td>一项不符扣 1 分</td><td></td></tr>
<tr><td>抽吸药液方法正确，不污染</td><td>4</td><td>一项不符扣 2 分</td><td></td></tr>
<tr><td>抽吸剂量准确，排尽空气，针头斜面向下，无浪费</td><td>4</td><td>一项不符扣 1 分</td><td></td></tr>
<tr><td>再次核对，置于无菌盘内备用</td><td>2</td><td>一项不符扣 1 分</td><td></td></tr>
<tr><td rowspan="12">注射</td><td rowspan="12">26</td><td>摆体位正确</td><td>2</td><td>一项不符扣 1 分</td><td></td></tr>
<tr><td>选择注射部位正确（并口述正确）</td><td>2</td><td>一项不符扣 2 分</td><td></td></tr>
<tr><td>消毒方法、范围（5 cm×5 cm）正确</td><td>2</td><td>一项不符扣 2 分</td><td></td></tr>
<tr><td>排尽空气，无浪费</td><td>2</td><td>一项不符扣 2 分</td><td></td></tr>
<tr><td>穿刺方法正确（进针角度：与穿刺皮肤呈 90°、深度正确），无污染</td><td>6</td><td>一项不符扣 2 分</td><td></td></tr>
<tr><td>固定方法正确，抽回血正确</td><td>4</td><td>一项不符扣 2 分</td><td></td></tr>
<tr><td>推注药物方法正确（缓慢推注，观察患者反应）</td><td>2</td><td>一项不符扣 1 分</td><td></td></tr>
<tr><td>拔针方法正确</td><td>2</td><td>一项不符扣 1 分</td><td></td></tr>
<tr><td>按压正确</td><td>2</td><td>一项不符扣 2 分</td><td></td></tr>
<tr><td>健康教育</td><td>2</td><td>一项不符扣 1 分</td><td></td></tr>
<tr><td colspan="4" style="display:none"></td></tr>
<tr><td colspan="4" style="display:none"></td></tr>
<tr><td rowspan="3">整理</td><td rowspan="3">8</td><td>患者卧位舒适，衣物整洁</td><td>2</td><td>一项不符扣 1 分</td><td></td></tr>
<tr><td>床单位整洁</td><td>2</td><td>一项不符扣 2 分</td><td></td></tr>
<tr><td>用物处理正确，7 步洗手法洗手，记录</td><td>4</td><td>一项不符扣 1 分</td><td></td></tr>
</table>

续表

<table>
<tr><th colspan="2">项　目</th><th>总分</th><th>技术操作要求</th><th>标准分</th><th>扣 分 说 明</th><th>得分</th></tr>
<tr><td rowspan="5">评价
22</td><td rowspan="3">熟练</td><td rowspan="3">10</td><td>操作轻稳、熟练、无菌观念强</td><td>4</td><td>一项不符扣 2 分</td><td></td></tr>
<tr><td>相关理论知识掌握熟练</td><td>2</td><td>酌情扣分</td><td></td></tr>
<tr><td>按规定时间完成(5 min),职业保护恰当</td><td>4</td><td>酌情扣分</td><td></td></tr>
<tr><td>效果</td><td>2</td><td>患者感觉安全舒适,无不良反应</td><td>2</td><td>酌情扣分</td><td></td></tr>
<tr><td>英语</td><td>10</td><td>发音标准,语言流畅,关爱患者,沟通良好</td><td>10</td><td>酌情扣分</td><td></td></tr>
<tr><td colspan="3">主考教师签字:</td><td>日期:</td><td colspan="2">总分:100</td><td>得分:</td></tr>
</table>

评分参考:91～100 分为优,81～90 分为良,71～80 分为中,60～70 分为差,低于 60 分为不及格。

注:1. 使用过期物品,该项考核为“不及格”。

2. 未核对患者或核对错误,该项考核为“不及格”。

3. 污染注射器乳头、针头而未考虑更换者,该项考核为“不及格”。

Chapter 11
Intravenous Infusion
静 脉 输 液

11.1 Peripheral Intravenous Infusion
周围静脉输液法

Purpose 操作目的

1. To provide adequate fluids and electrolytes to maintain the balance of body fluid and electrolyte.

补充人体需要的液体、电解质，以维持水、电解质平衡。

2. To increase circulation blood volume in order to improve microcirculation and maintain blood pressure.

增加循环血量，改善微循环及维持血压。

3. To provide nutrition for tissue regeneration, weight gain and maintenance of nitrogen balance.

供给营养物质，促进组织修复，增加体重，维持正氮平衡。

4. To treat disease by administering intravenous medication.

经静脉输入药物治疗疾病。

Assessment 评估

1. Assess the patient's age, level of consciousness, health condition, cardiac,

pulmonary and renal function, allergy history and purpose of intravenous infusion.

评估患者的年龄、意识、病情、心肺功能及肾功能、过敏史及静脉输液目的。

2. Assess the patient's veins, skin of venipuncture site and mobility status of the limb.

评估患者的静脉穿刺部位皮肤情况及肢体活动度。

3. Assess the patient's psychological status, ability to cooperate, communication skills, understanding of intravenous infusion and its plan.

评估患者的心理状态、合作程度、表达能力、对静脉输液及输液计划的了解程度。

Gather Equipment 物品准备

治疗盘内:prescribed medication 医嘱用药,sterile saline 无菌生理盐水,metal file 砂轮,sterile gauzes 无菌纱布,sheath 瓶套,antiseptic solution 消毒液,sterile swabs 无菌棉签,tourniquet 止血带,sterile drape 无菌治疗巾,syringes 注射器,disposable infusion set 一次性输液器,medical infusion fixation paster 输液贴,infusion lable 输液标签,infusion card 输液卡,adhesion tape 胶布。

治疗盘外:prescription chart 医嘱单,kidney basin 弯盘,small pillow 小枕,hand sanitizer 洗手液,IV stand/pole 输液架,sharp container 锐器盒。

Procedure 操作过程

1. Report and tidy your dress.

报告并整理仪表。

2. Check the validity of hand sanitizer and wash hands in 7 steps and put on the mask.

检查洗手液的有效期,7 步洗手法洗手并戴口罩。

3. Gather equipments, assemble the solution and medication according to the prescription chart, and check for the prescription and equipments.

备齐用物,准备输液溶液及药物,核对医嘱及用品。

4. Check the solution and medications for color, clarity and expiration date. Observe the solution bag/bottle for chasms or leaks.

检查输液溶液及药液的颜色、澄清度及有效期。观察输液袋/瓶有无裂痕或漏液。

5. Type or fill the patient's name, bed number and the prescription in the infusion cards according to doctor's order.

根据医嘱，打印或填写输液卡，包括患者床号、姓名及医嘱内容。

6. Lable the solution bag/bottle with the infusion card.

在输液袋上贴上标签。

7. Remove the protective cap of the solution bottle. Put a sheath over the glass bottle.

揭去输液袋的保护盖，给输液瓶套上瓶套。

8. Clean the surface of rubber seal with antiseptic swabs routinely and allow it to dry.

使用无菌棉签常规消毒瓶塞，待干。

9. Ensure that the medication and solution are compatible, then withdraw the correct dosage of medication.

确保药物与溶液没有配伍禁忌，然后抽吸准确剂量的药液。

10. Add the prescription medications into the bag/bottle, check the solution for color and clarity once again. Make sure that the solution is clear and contains no particles or precipitates.

按医嘱加入药物，再次检查溶液的颜色及澄清度，确保输液溶液澄清、无颗粒及沉淀物。

11. Clean the surface of rubber seal with an alcohol swabs once again if necessary.

必要时用酒精棉签再次消毒瓶塞。

12. Select an infusion set, check its expiration date and integrity, and open the set.

选择输液器，检查有效期及完整性，打开输液器。

13. Move the roller clamp to "off" position.

关闭输液器调节器。

14. Remove the protector caps from the spikes of infusion set, keep spikes uncontaminated, and insert the spikes through the rubber seal into the port of solution bag/bottle thoroughly.

取下输液器的输液管或通气管针头的保护帽，保持针头无菌，将针头经胶塞全部插入输液袋/瓶内。

15. Cover the medical waste and garbage bin, wash hands and remove the mask.

盖上污物桶(医用垃圾桶、生活垃圾桶)盖，洗手、摘口罩。

16. Take the equipment to the ward. Assess the working environment.

携用物至病室内。评估操作环境。

17. Check the patient's bed number and name. Explain the purpose of the

operation and getting cooperation from the patient.

核对床头卡上床号和患者姓名。解释操作目的，取得患者合作。

18. Open the cap of medical waste and garbage bin, wash hands and put on the mask.

打开污物桶（医用垃圾桶、生活垃圾桶）盖，洗手、戴口罩。

19. Check the medication against prescription chart.

根据医嘱单核对药物的名称。

20. Confirm that the patient has emptied bladder or bowel.

确定患者已排空大小便。

21. Hang up the solution bag/bottle upside-down on the IV pole.

将输液袋/瓶倒挂于输液架上。

22. Compress Muphy's drip chamber and release, allowing it to fill one-half to two-thirds full.

挤压莫菲滴管后放松，使液面达到 1/2～2/3。

23. Hold the winged needle with one hand facing the basin, release the roller clamp slowly with the other hand, to allow solution to travel from the drip chamber through the tubing to the tip of the winged needle.

一手持头皮针朝向弯盘，另一只手慢慢放松调节器，使药液从滴管顺着输液管流到头皮针针尖。

24. After the tubing and winged needle are primed, return the roller clamp to "off" position.

输液管及头皮针充满药液后，将调节器调至"关"的位置。

25. Check the entire length of the tubing and winged needle, tap the infusion tubing where air bubbles are located if necessary, to ensure that the whole tubing is clear of air.

检查整条输液管及头皮针，必要时弹击输液管内停留的气泡，确保整条输液管没有空气。

26. Place the winged needle into the medication tray.

将头皮针放到治疗盘里。

27. Assist the patient to comfortable position.

协助患者取舒适体位。

28. Place a tourniquet 10-15 cm above the proposes venipuncture site.

在穿刺点上方 10～15 cm 处扎止血带。

29. Select a well-dilated vein for IV insertion distally to proximally.

从远端到近端选择充盈的静脉。

30. Put a small pillow under the venipuncture site selected if necessary.

必要时在所选择的静脉穿刺部位下垫小枕。

31. Loosen the tourniquet.

松开止血带。

32. Clean the venipuncture site about 8 cm × 10 cm with antiseptic swabs routinely, and allow it to dry.

常规消毒静脉穿刺部位皮肤约 8 cm×10 cm，待干。

33. Open the package of medical infusion fixation paster, and place it within tray.

撕开医用输液贴外包装，放于治疗盘内。

34. Place a tourniquet 10-15 cm above the proposes venipuncture site.

在穿刺点上方 10～15 cm 处扎止血带。

35. Clean the venipuncture sit again.

再次消毒穿刺部位皮肤。

36. Recheck the patient's name, solution and medication. Make sure that the whole tubing is clear of air bubbles.

再次核对患者、溶液及药名，并确保整条输液管内无气泡。

37. Remove the protective cap from the winged needle.

取下头皮针的针头帽。

38. Expel air once again.

再次排气。

39. If a dorsal vein of hand is selected, ask the patient to clench a fist.

如选择手背静脉，嘱患者握拳。

40. Place the thumb of your nondominant hand below the selected vein and put the skin taut to stabilize the vein. With the needle bevel facing up, insert the needle at a 15°-30° angle through skin over the selected vein or along the site of the vein, then follow course of the vein and enter the vein.

一手拇指绷紧静脉下端皮肤以固定静脉。针尖斜面向上，与皮肤呈 15°～30°角自静脉上方或侧方刺入皮下，再沿静脉走向滑行刺入静脉。

41. When blood flows back into the tubing of the winged needle, carefully advance the needle up course of the vein a little further.

见头皮针管内有回血，再顺静脉走行进针少许。

42. Release the tourniquet and ask the patient to release fist.

松止血带，嘱患者松拳。

43. Open the clamp.

打开调节器。

44. Observe the drip chamber for fluid flow.

观察滴管内液体滴入的情况。

45. If fluid flows easily and there's no sudden swelling and no pain at the venipuncture site, secure the needle well with medical infusion fixation paster. Loop the tubing connecting to the needle and secure it with taps.

如果液体滴入顺畅,静脉注射局部无肿胀、无疼痛,则用输液贴妥善固定针头。将针头附近的输液管环绕后用胶布固定。

46. Immobilize the joint in functional position with a splint if necessary.

必要时用夹板固定关节于功能位。

47. Adjust the flow rate as ordered or according to the patient's age, health condition and medication property. In general, 40-60 gtt/min is set for adults, and 20-40 gtt/min for children.

按医嘱或根据患者的年龄、病情及药液性质调节输液滴速。一般情况成年人 40～60 滴/分,儿童 20～40 滴/分。

48. Write down the date, time and flow rate on the infusion card at bedside, and sign on the card.

在患者床边的输液卡上记录输液的日期、时间及滴速并签名。

49. Recheck the patient's name, bed number, solution and medication.

再次核对患者的姓名、床号、输液溶液及药名。

50. Tell the patient not to adjust the flow rate.

交代患者不要自行调节滴速。

51. Instruct the patient how to move without dislodging the IV needle.

指导患者活动的方法以防止针头脱出。

52. Remove the tourniquet and the pillow, assist the patient to comfortable position and tidy up the bed. Discard all used equipment appropriately.

取出止血带和小枕,协助患者取舒适体位,整体床单位。清理用物。

53. Observe the venipuncture site, flow rate and the patient's response periodically.

定时观察静脉穿刺部位、滴速及患者的反应。

Nurse Alert 护理事项

1. Follow the checking procedure, use aseptic techniques strictly.

严格执行查对制度及无菌技术。

2. Dispense medications to solutions and prioritize the infusion solution according to the patient's health condition and medication property.

根据病情及药物性质合理分配药物及安排输液顺序。

3. Select an appropriate venipuncture site according to the patient's health condition and medication property. Area should be free of lesions or scars and away from joints and venous valves or bifurcation.

根据病情及药物性质选择合适的静脉穿刺部位。避免在皮肤受损、瘢痕处进针，避开关节和静脉瓣或静脉分叉处。

4. Regulate intravenous flow rate correctly.

准确调节输液速度。

5. Observe the patient frequently.

经常巡视患者。

6. Observe the patient for infusion reaction and instruct the patient to report any symptoms and signs of shortness of breath, chest pain, or skin reaction such as itching and rashes.

观察患者有无输液反应，并指导患者如有气促、胸痛和皮肤瘙痒、皮疹等皮肤反应要及时回报。

New Words and Expressions

单 词 表

intravenous [ˌintrəˈviːnəs] *adj*. 静脉内的

infusion [inˈfjuːʒən] *n*. 输入液体，灌入液体

peripheral [pəˈrifərəl] *adj*. 外周的

electrolyte [iˈlektrəˌlait] *n*. 电解质；电解质类

nitrogen [ˈnaitrədʒən] *n*. [化学]氮

allergy [ˈælədʒiː] *n*. 过敏性反应

venipuncture [ˈveniˌpʌŋktʃə] *n*. 静脉穿刺

metal file 砂轮

antiseptic [ˌæntiˈseptik] *n*. 防腐剂，抗菌剂

tourniquet [ˈtuənikit] *n*. [外科] 止血带；压脉器；压血带

sharp [ʃɑːp] *adj*. 尖锐的

Communication Model
沟通模板

Self-introduction Model 常规介绍模板

Good morning/afternoon teachers, my name is ××, I come from class ××, my student's number is ××. Today, I am going to show you the process of intravenous infusion, the equipments I have prepared are ... ,everything is ready, may I start?

早上/下午好老师,我的名字是××,来自××班,我的学号是××。今天,我要展示的操作是静脉输液,所准备的用物有……,准备完毕,请求开始。

Assessment 评估

The ward is tidy and well ventilated. There is no patient receiving therapy or dining.

病室整洁通风良好,没有患者进餐或接受治疗。

Communication 沟通

Good morning, sir. May I have your name ? OK,Mr ××, I'm your duty nurse, how are you feeling today? It is time for you to have the intravenous infusion now. Have you used ×× before? It can (prevent/treat infection, fall blood pressure, decrease blood sugar, increase blood volume, release pain ...). It is good for your health. (If the drug is penicillin, your allergy testing result must be negative.)

早上好,先生。请告诉我您的名字好吗?好的,××先生,我是您的责任护士,今天感觉如何?现在要为您进行静脉输液。您以前用过××吗?这种药可以(预防/治疗感染,降血压,降血糖,增加血容量,缓解疼痛……)。它对您的健康有好处。(如果该药物是青霉素,您的过敏实验结果必须是阴性的。)

The procedure will take a long time. Do you want to go to the washroom first?

这个过程需要很长时间,您需要先去洗手间吗?

Check the patient and medication according to the doctor's order.

根据医嘱核对患者及药物。

Bed number 5, Robert Walker. Normal saline, concentration is 0.9%. The dosage is 250 mL, expiration date is December 5, 2011. There is no particles and precipitates. The drug is effective and it can be used.

5号床，罗伯特·沃克。生理盐水，浓度是0.9%。剂量是250 mL，有效日期是2011年12月5日。无杂质和沉淀。该药物是有效的，可以使用。

Selecting a vein　选择静脉

Mr ××, which hand for you is convenient/comfortable/available /suitable for IV? Left hand or right? May I see your hand? May I see your vein? Please roll up your sleeves and clench your fist. Do you feel pain when I press here? OK, that is in good condition. So don't be nervous, I'm in good hands.

先生，哪只手比较方便/舒适/可用/适合静脉输液手？左手还是右手？我可以看一下你的手吗？我可以看看你的静脉吗？请卷起你的袖子，握紧你的拳头。我压这儿的时候你觉得痛吗？好吧，血管的条件良好，请不要紧张，相信我，我扎得特别好！

Second Check　二次核对

Mr ××, right? OK. I'm going to have a injection for you, don't be nervous / please calm down/relax/take it easy.

××先生，对吗？好了，我要进针了，别紧张/镇定点儿/放松/放轻松。

Inserting the needle　穿刺

Do you feel pain? OK, release your fist, the solution flow smoothly.

你觉得疼吗？放松拳头，药液流得很顺利。

Adjusting the flow rate　调节滴速

Please do not adjust the flow rate by yourself/ Please do not touch the roller clamp. Keep stay on the bed for 30 minutes at least.

请不要擅自调节滴速/请不要触碰流量调节阀。在床上待30 min以上。

Third check　三次核对

Would you like to tell me your name again? Thank you, Mr ××, if you feel any uncomfortable, don't hesitate to call me/please press the button on the call signal, and I will come here to help you. Don't be worried, you will be recover soon after the treatment.

请再告诉我您的名字？谢谢您，××先生，如果您有任何不舒服，不要不好意思叫我/请按呼叫器上的按钮，我会来帮助您的。不要担心，治疗后您将会很快康复的。

Remove the needle　拔针

I'm coming now. Do you feel much better now? The infusion is finished. Dose it hurt? Very good. You are a brave boy/girl. Do not forget to take the medical following the doctor's order. Everything will be fine. Have a good rest!

我又来了。你现在感觉好多了吗？药液输完了。痛吗？真棒，你是一个勇敢的男孩/女孩。不要忘记遵照医嘱服药。你会好起来的。好好休息吧！

Scoring Criteria 16
评分细则 16

项目		总分	技术操作要求	标准分	扣分说明	得分
评估 12	仪表	4	仪表端庄、服装整洁、修剪指甲、洗手、戴口罩	4	一项不符扣2分	
	物品	4	物品备齐，治疗车上、下放置合理	4	一项不符扣2分	
	环境		环境符合要求			
	患者	4	了解患者病情、意识状态及合作程度、局部皮肤情况、血管状况，是否有排尿、便的需要	4	一项不符扣1分	
实施 68	准备药液	4	正确核对、检查药液	2	一项不符扣2分	
			正确填写输液卡、瓶签	2	一项不符扣2分	
	核对解释	8	适时三查七对，内容全面（药物、患者、床头卡共同核对）	6	每次查对不符各扣2分	
			根据病情解释（操作目的、过程、配合方法）	2	一项不符扣1分	
	输液	44	药瓶消毒过程正确，检查、取用、连接输液器正确	4	一项不符扣2分	
			输液架高度适宜	1	一项不符扣1分	
			一次排气成功，滴管液面高度合适，不浪费药液	3	一项不符扣1分	
			垫巾放置合理，合理选择血管（口述）	3	一项不符扣2分	
			皮肤消毒范围正确	4	一项不符扣1分	
			待干，准备胶布，放置合理	4	一项不符扣2分	
			再次消毒	2	一项不符扣2分	
			二次排气成功，不浪费药液	4	一项不符扣2分	
			二次核对	2	一项不符扣2分	
			静脉穿刺方法正确（进针角度、深度）	4	一项不符扣2分	
			穿刺后及时三松（松拳、松止血带、松调节器）	3	一项不符扣1分	
			胶布适时准备，放置合理，固定牢固、美观	2	一项不符扣1分	
			根据病情确定输液滴速，正确调节滴速	2	一项不符扣2分	
			三次核对	4	一项不符扣2分	
			正确填写巡视卡	1	一项不符扣1分	
			合理健康教育（勿自调滴速，保护针眼，药物使用注意事项）	3	一项不符扣1分	
	拔针	6	关闭（调小）调节阀，揭胶布手法轻柔，拔针手法正确，按压针眼及时	6	一项不符扣2分	
	整理	6	患者卧位舒适，衣物整洁，床单位整洁	2	一项不符扣2分	
			用物处理正确，洗手，记录	4	一项不符扣2分	

续表

项	目	总分	技术操作要求	标准分	扣分说明	得分
评价 22	熟练	10	操作轻稳、熟练、无菌观念强	4	一项不符扣 2 分	
			相关理论知识掌握熟练	2	一项不符扣 2 分	
			按规定时间完成(12 min),职业保护恰当	4	每超过 30 s 扣 1 分	
	效果	2	患者感觉安全舒适,无不良反应	2	酌情扣分	
	英语	10	发音标准,语言流畅,关爱患者,沟通良好	10	酌情扣分	
主考教师签字:			日期:	总分:100	得分:	

评分参考:91～100 分为优,81～90 分为良,71～80 分为中,60～70 分为差,低于 60 分为不及格。

注:1. 出现下列情况之一者该项考核为“不及格”:使用过期物品,未核对患者或核对错误,输液器针头污染未更换,局部皮肤污染未重新消毒。

2. 其他违反无菌原则的行为 1 次扣总分 4 分。

Chapter 12

CPR（Cardiopulmonary Resuscitation）心肺复苏术

Purpose　操作目的

CPR is an emergency lifesaving procedure that is performed when a person's own breathing or heartbeat have stopped, such as in cases of trauma, poisoning, electric shock, heart attack, or drowning. CPR combines rescue breathing and chest compressions. Rescue breathing provides oxygen to the person's lungs. Chest compressions keep oxygen-rich blood circulating until an effective heartbeat and breathing can be restored. Permanent brain damage or death can occur within minutes if a person's blood flow stops. Permanent brain damage begins after only 4 minutes without oxygen, and death can occur as soon as 4 - 6 minutes later.

Therefore, you must start these procedures as early as possible.

心肺复苏是对由于外伤、中毒、电击、心脏病发作或淹溺等各种原因导致的呼吸、心跳停止而采取的紧急生命抢救过程。CPR 包括重建呼吸功能及胸部按压。重建呼吸功能为患者提供气体交换。胸部按压可以在心跳及呼吸功能有效恢复之前维持患者血液循环。患者血液循环停止后数分钟可造成脑部不可逆性的损伤或死亡。脑部不可逆性的损伤在缺氧 4 min 后开始，而死亡通常发生在 4～6 min 之后。

因此，心肺复苏的实施过程越早越好。

Symptoms　症状

no breathing or difficulty breathing (gasping)　呼吸停止或呼吸困难

no pulse 大动脉搏动消失

unconsciousness 意识丧失

dilated pupils 瞳孔散大

pale or cyanosis 皮肤苍白或发绀

no heartbeat and heart sound 心脏搏动或心音消失

no bleeding 伤口不出血

Procedure 操作过程

1. See someone falling on the ground.

看到有人倒地。

2. Confirm the safety of environment.

确认现场环境安全。

3. Check for responsiveness: Shake or tap the person gently. See if the person moves or response to you. Shout: "Are you OK?" Check for the pulse of carotid artery and place your ear close to the person's mouth and nose in 10 seconds. Watch for chest movement. Feel for breath on your cheek. If the person has normal breathing, coughing, or movement, do not begin chest compressions. Doing so may cause the heart to stop beating. If there are no response, no pulse and no breathing, call for help immediately.

判断意识:轻轻摇动或轻拍患者,观察患者是否挪动或做出反应。大声呼叫:"喂,你怎么了?"在 10 s 内检查患者颈动脉搏动并将耳朵贴近患者口鼻,观察胸壁活动,用脸颊感觉患者呼吸。观察胸廓起伏。如果患者存在正常呼吸,咳嗽或肢体活动,不要为患者实施心脏按压,否则会造成心脏停搏。如果患者无任何反应,无动脉搏动及自主呼吸,立即呼救。

4. If you have help, tell one person to call 120 while begins CPR. If you are alone, begin chest compression for 30 times and then call 120 by yourself, after that continue CPR.

周围有人请大声呼救,告诉旁边的人拨打 120 并立即实施 CPR。如果周围没有人,马上实施心脏按压 30 下后自己拨打 120,之后继续 CPR 程序。

5. Carefully place the person on their back. If there is a chance the person has a spinal injury, you should move the person carefully to prevent the head and neck from twisting.

小心置患者于仰卧位。如果患者存在脊柱受伤的危险,应小心挪动患者,防止头、颈部转动。

6. Open his/her clothes and trouser belt.

解开患者上衣及裤带。

7. Perform chest compressions: Place the heel of one hand on the breastbone—right between the nipples. Place the heel of your other hand on top of the first hand. Position your body directly over your hands. Give chest compressions for 30 times. These compressions should be fast and hard and rhythm no less than 100 times per minute. Press down more than 5 cm into the chest.

心脏按压:将一只手的掌跟放于两乳头中央的胸骨处,将另一掌跟放于第一只手上。操作者身体直立于手掌之上进行 30 次的胸外按压。按压应快速而有力,节律至少 100 次/分。胸骨下陷至少 5 cm 后使胸廓扩张。

8. Open the airway: Lift up the chin with two fingers. At the same time, tilt the head by pushing down on the forehead with the other hand.

开放气道:用两个手指抬举患者的下颌,同时另一只手压低前额。

9. Mouth to mouth breathing: If the person is not breathing or has trouble breathing, cover their mouth tightly with your mouth. Pinch the nose closed, keep the chin lifted and head tilted, and give two rescue breaths. Each breath should take about a second and make the chest rise.

口对口人工呼吸:如果患者没有呼吸或呼吸困难,双唇紧紧包住患者双唇,捏紧鼻孔,保持使患者下颌抬高、前额向下倾斜进行吹气两次。每次吹气持续数秒钟使患者胸壁抬高。

10. Give the person 2 more breaths. The chest should rise.

继续吹两大口气,使胸廓扩张。

11. Continue CPR 30 chest compressions followed by 2 breaths, then repeat for 5 times or until the person recovers or help arrives.

反复进行 2 次人工呼吸跟随 30 次按压的复苏操作 5 轮或直到患者恢复或帮助的人出现。

12. Recheck the pulse of carotid artery and breath for 10 seconds.

再次判断经动脉搏动和呼吸 10 s。

13. State the signs of effective CPR.

陈述心肺复苏有效指征。

14. Doing psychological nursing care to patient while helping his/her to wear clothes.

边为患者穿好衣服边对患者进行心理安慰。

Nurse Alert 护理事项

1. Rescue the patient on supine position and avoid moving a lot to delay the save time.

患者仰卧进行抢救，避免因搬动而延误时机。

2. Remove oropharyngeal secretions and foreign bodies, keep airway opening. Pay attention that the most common cause of respiratory resuscitation failure is respiratory tract obstruction and mouth-to-mouth contact is lax. Because of the respiratory tract obstruction, the tongue have played an important role as a valve, only let air into the stomach but don't let it eliminate from the stomach. It can cause severe stomach expansion, and elevate diaphragmatic muscle to hinder the ventilation. Being Worse, it can cause a stomach contents reflux and make the patient in the risk of inhalation of stomach contents.

清除口咽分泌物、异物，保证气道通畅。注意呼吸复苏失败的最常见原因是呼吸道阻塞和口对口接触不严。由于呼吸道阻塞，舌头起到了活瓣作用，只让空气压进胃内，不让空气再由胃排出，造成严重的胃扩张，可使膈肌显著升高，阻碍充分的通气。更甚者或造成胃内容物反流，造成将呕吐物吸入的危险。

3. Pressing point must be correct and press in the right way to prevent the fracture of sternum and ribs. It is forbidden to press on the sternal angle and xiphoid and the chest.

按压部位要准确，方法正确，以防止胸骨、肋骨骨折。严禁按压胸骨角、剑突下及左右胸部。

4. Doing mouth-to-mouth breathing and chest compressions simultaneously. Breathing should be in intermittent of compressions. Do not press the chest in the situation of lung inflation to avoid damaging the lungs and reducing ventilation effect.

人工呼吸和胸外心脏按压同时进行。吹气应在放松按压的间歇进行。肺充气时，不可按压胸部，以免损伤肺部，降低通气效果。

New Words and Expressions
单 词 表

cardiopulmonary [ˌkɑːdiəuˈpulmən(ə)ri] *adj.* 心肺的

resuscitation [riˌsʌsiˈteiʃən] *n.* 复苏

trauma [ˈtrɔːmə] *n.* 创伤
drowning [ˈdrauniŋ] *n.* 溺死
compression [kəmˈpreʃən] *n.* 压迫
rescue [ˈreskjuː] *n.* 营救;援救;解救
circulating [ˈsəːkjuleitiŋ] *v.* 循环(circulate 的 ing 形式)
restored [riˈstɔːd] *v.* 修复(restore 的过去式);恢复健康
dilated [daiˈleitid] *adj.* 扩大的;膨胀的
cyanosis [ˌsaiəˈnəusis] *n.* 苍白病;发绀
spinal [ˈspainəl] *adj.* 脊柱的
twisting [twist] *n.* 扭转 *adj.* 转动的
nipple [ˈnipəl] *n.* 乳头
rhythm [ˈriðəm] *n.* 节奏;韵律
pinch [pintʃ] *vt.* 捏;挤压

Communication Model
沟通模板

Self-introduction Model 常规介绍模板

Good morning/afternoon teachers, my name is ××, I come from class ××, my student's number is ××. Today, I am going to show you the process of CPR. The equipment I have to prepare are two pieces of gauzes. Everything is ready, may I start?

早上/下午好老师,我的名字是××,来自××班,我的学号是××。今天,我要展示的操作是心肺复苏。我准备的物品有两块纱布。准备完毕,请求开始。

Assessment 评估

The patient was collapsed on the ground. He may suffer from cardiac arrest. Cardiac arrest means that there is no blood flow through the body, and the patient will die within minutes unless we give him CPR as soon as possible. Now, I will show you the process.

患者突然倒地,他可能出现心搏骤停。心搏骤停的意思是血流停止,如果不为患者实施救治在几分钟内患者将会死亡。现在,我要为您示范救治过程。

The area is safe and it is suitable to do the CPR for the patient.

现场环境安全,适合为患者实施心肺复苏。

Check for responsiveness, tap the patient's shoulder and shout loudly: "Hello, sir! Are you OK? Can you hear me?"

判断意识,轻拍患者肩膀,大声呼唤:"先生您好,您怎么了? 您还好吗? 能听到我说话吗?"

Check for carotid artery pulsation and breathing for 1-10 seconds: one to ten. Assess if the thoracic go ups and downs, the gas overflow from mouth and nose, carotid pulse has disappeared. (The patient is no pulse and no breathing).

判断颈动脉搏动及呼吸 1～10 s,判断胸廓有无起伏,口鼻有无气体溢出,颈动脉搏动是否消失。(口述:患者无脉搏及呼吸)

Waving for help: "Help, someone help! Please call the 120!" Or call 120 by yourself: "Hello, is this 120 Emergency Center?" (Hello, this is 120 command and dispatch center, what can I do for you?) Here is..., someone was collapsed on the ground, and his heart and breathing may stop, please come here as soon as possible! Thank you.

挥手呼救:"来人啊,救命啊,请帮我拨打 120。"或自己拨打:"您好,是 120 急救中心吗?"(您好,这里是 120 急救中心,很高兴为您服务。)这里是××,有人突然倒地,他的心跳和呼吸骤停,请尽快过来救治,谢谢。

Chest compressions: One ... thirty.

胸部按压:1……30 下。

Open the airway and take mouth to mouth breathing: two breathing.

开放气道及口对口人工呼吸:2 次呼吸。

Do the same process for five times.

做 5 遍同样的过程。

Recheck the patient　再次检查患者

The pluse reappear, breathing recover, pupil contracted, the colour of the face, lips, and nail bed from purplish to ruddy/rosy. All of this indicates the resuscitation is successful, we can give the patient advanced life-support treatment.

患者大动脉搏动出现,自主呼吸出现,瞳孔由散大变缩小,面色、口唇、甲床由发绀变为红润。所有体征表明心肺复苏抢救成功,我们为患者提供高级生命支持。

Psychological communication　心理护理

Hi, sir, you are awake! I'm a nurse. You have suffered from cardiac arrest, but

you are safe now. Your wife is beside you. Don't worry, the ambulance is coming, I will sent you to the hospital. Please relax for a while. I will be here with you till the personnel is coming.

先生,您好,您终于醒了。我是一名护士。您刚出现了心搏骤停,但是现在您安全了。您的妻子就在您的身边,不要担心,急救车已经在路上了,我会送您到医院,稍事休息一会吧,我会在医务人员到来前一直陪在您身边的。

New Words and Expressions
单 词 表

pupil [ˈpjuːpəl] *n.* 瞳孔
contracted [kənˈtræktid] *adj.* 收缩了的;狭小的
purplish [ˈpəːpliʃ] *adj.* 略带紫色的
ruddy [ˈrʌdi] *adj.* 红的;红润的
rosy [ˈrəuziː] *adj.* 蔷薇色的,玫瑰红色的
advanced [ədˈvɑːnst] *adj.* 先进的;高级的
cardiac [ˈkɑːdiˌæk] *adj.* 心脏的;心脏病的
arrest [əˈrest] *vt.* 逮捕;阻止
ambulance [ˈæmbjuləns] *n.* 救护车
personnel [ˌpəːsəˈnel] *n.* 人员

Scoring Criteria 17
评分细则 17

项 目		总分	技术操作要求	标准分	扣 分 说 明	得分
准备 6	仪表	4	仪表端庄、服装整洁、修剪指甲、洗手、戴口罩	4	一项不符扣 1 分	
	物品	2	准备纱布两块，硬木板(必要时)	2	一项不符扣 1 分	
实施 72	报告	2	介绍自己及即将演示的操作	2	一项不符扣 1 分	
	评估	2	评估现场环境是否安全(采用动作及语言表现)	2	一项不符扣 1 分	
	C	30	抢救者双腿分开，一条腿的膝盖对着患者的肩头，另一条腿的膝盖对着患者的肚脐	2	一项不符扣 1 分	
			判断意识：轻拍重唤	4	一项不符扣 2 分	
			判断脉搏和呼吸体位及姿势正确(大声数 1～10 s)	4	一项不符扣 2 分	
			抢救者向周围人群求助，没有帮助者需自己拨打 120，进入抢救状态	2	一项不符扣 2 分	
			将患者放置复苏体位：患者仰卧于硬木板上或地板上	2	一项不符扣 2 分	
			解开上衣及腰带，暴露胸部，选择按压部位方法正确	4	一项不符扣 2 分	
			姿势：手掌掌根放在按压处，另一手抓住着力点的手，手指上翘，掌根贴近胸骨用力按压。抢救者双臂绷紧，双肩在患者胸骨正上方，按压过程中双手位置放置正确	8	一项不符扣 2 分	
			垂直向下用力按压，按压有力，不间断。按压与放松的时间大致相等，按压放松时胸廓充分回缩、膨胀；按压深度为胸骨下陷 5 cm；按压频率大于 100 次/分，口念任何有帮助的数字(需要读出声音)，按压 30 次	4	一项不符扣 1 分	
	A	8	开放气道 1. 检查口腔，如有呼吸道分泌物或异物应及时清除；如有义齿应取出 2. 任选一种方法开放气道，垫纱布	8	一项不符扣 4 分	
	B	8	捏住患者的鼻孔，保持气道开放状态，给予患者通气 2 次，每次通气 1 s，吹气量为 500～1000 mL/次，可见胸廓明显起伏	8	一项不符扣 2 分	
	循环	22	重新定位按压点并开放气道，完成 30 次按压，2 次通气	8	一项不符扣 2 分	
			口述做五个循环	2	一项不符扣 2 分	
			复苏后评价：判断脉搏和呼吸 10 s 口述复苏成功有效指标(至少四项)	6	第一项扣 2 分 第二项扣 4 分	
			整理患者衣物，安慰并给予心理支持，拿走纱布	6	一项不符扣 2 分	

续表

项目		总分	技术操作要求	标准分	扣分说明	得分
评价 22	熟练	8	操作熟练、步骤合理	4	酌情扣分	
			按规定时间完成(3 min)	4	每过 30 s 扣 1 分	
	效果	4	表现力良好,能营造紧张的抢救气氛	4	酌情扣分	
	英语	10	发音标准,语言流畅,关爱患者,沟通良好	10	酌情扣分	
主考教师签字:			日期:	总分:100	得分:	

评分参考:91～100 分为优,81～90 分为良,71～80 分为中,60～70 分为差,低于 60 分为不及格。

Appendix
Nursing Shift Reports
附录
护士交班报告

1. Head nurse morning report

Good morning, everyone, today is January 13, 2013. Yesterday there were 36 patients originally, 9 patients were admitted, 7 patients were discharged. The number of patients now in our ward is 38.

Yesterday selective coronary angiography was performed in 11 patients, 3 patients for PCI. Electrophysiological examination and radiofrequency ablation was performed in 3 patients, 1 for atrial fibrillation, another 2 for paroxysmal supraventricular tachycardia. All the puncture sites of operation recovered well and other patients in our ward were stable.

That is all, thanks.

Head nurse:Jin ling

1. 护士长晨会报告

大家早上好,今天是 2013 年 1 月 13 日。昨日原有病例 36 人,新入院 9 人,7 人出院,目前病室患者数为 38 人。

昨天 11 人做了选择性冠状动脉造影,3 人进行 PCI(经皮冠状动脉介入治疗)。3 人进行电生理检查及射频消融术,1 人出现房颤,2 人出现阵发性室上性心动过速。所有患者的术后切口恢复均较好,病室内其他患者病情平稳。

就这些,谢谢。

护士长:金玲

2. Nursing shift reports in daytime

There are 33 patients today, 2 patients were admitted, 1 patient was shifted in, 5 patients were discharged. The total number of patients in our ward is 31.

Bed No 4, Libo, male, 60 years old. He had palpitations for 4 years and felt serious for 6 months, He was admitted in July 10, 2012. He was diagnosed as paroxysmal atrial fibrillation and performed radiofrequency of CPVI successfully in July 10, 2012. The patient felt dizziness with nausea emesis all day in yesterday, but no anepia limb action disorders and conscious disturbance, We invited neural physician to check the patient at once, the doctor suggested to perform head CT and TCD check tomorrow morning, At present the doctor suggested to intravenous infusion gastrodine and intramuscular injection promethazine therapy. This morning the condition of the patient is stable.

Yesterday electrophysiological examination and radiofrequency ablation were performed in 2 patients and one for AF and the other one for paroxysmal supraventricular tachycardia. All the arteries and veins recovered successfully and other patients in our ward were stable.

That is all, thanks.

Duty nurse: Liu ying

2. 日间护士交班报告

今日原有患者总数 33 人,新入院 2 人,1 人转科,5 人出院。现有患者总数为 31 人。

4 床,李博,男,60 岁。4 年前出现心悸,近 6 个月感觉加重。于 2012 年 7 月 10 日入院。诊断为阵发性心房颤动并于入院当天成功实施 CPVI 射频消融术。昨日患者感觉眩晕并伴恶心呕吐,但是不伴失语性肢体活动障碍和意识障碍。我们立即请神经科医生会诊。医生建议次晨实施头部 CT 和 TCD 检查。目前医生建议静脉输注天麻素,肌内注射异丙嗪治疗。今晨患者一般状态良好。

昨日共有两人接受电生理检查及射频消融术,一个是房颤患者,另一个是阵发性室上性心动过速。目前病室内其他患者病情平稳,静脉及动脉条件恢复较好。

就这些,谢谢。

责任护士:刘瑛

3. Nursing shift reports on night

Yesterday there were 32 patients, 4 patients were admitted, 1 patients were shifted in, 4 patients were discharged. The number of patients in our ward is 33.

Bed No7, Zhang xiuling, female, 64 years old, she had palpitations for 7 years. She was diagnosed as paroxysmal atrial fibrillation. The patient saddened for palpitations with chest tightness, shortness of breath at 18:54 last night. After examination of ECG at once, she was diagnosed as atrial fibrillation. After given amiodarone 300 mg (milligram) venous transfusion, the patient has recovered sinus rhythm at 19:30 last night, At present the patient is stable.

Yesterday there were 6 patients underwent PTCA (percutaneous transcoronary angioplasty) and 1 patient underwent radio frequency. Their condition was stable all night.

The other patients in our ward were all stable.

That is all, thanks.

Duty nurse: Zhang ming

3. 夜班护士交班报告

昨日原有患者32人，新入院4人，1人转科，4人出院，现有患者总数为33人。7床，张秀玲，女，64岁。7年前出现心悸，入院诊断为阵发性心房颤动。患者于昨晚18点54分因心悸、胸闷、气短感到伤心难过。立即为患者实施心电图检查，心电图显示房颤。经静脉输注胺碘酮300 mg后患者于19点30分恢复窦性心律。目前患者一般状态平稳。

昨日有6人接受PTCA(经皮冠状动脉成形术)治疗，1人接受射频消融术。患者整晚状态平稳。

其他患者状态平稳。

就这些，谢谢。

责任护士：张明

参考文献

References

[1] 李小寒，尚少梅. 基础护理学. [M]. 5 版. 北京：人民卫生出版社，2012.

[2] 徐萍. 基础护理学实训指导[M]. 西安：西安交通大学出版社，2011.

[3] 万丽红. 基础护理学基本技能[M]. 广州：广东科技出版社，2009.

[4] 王文秀，王颖. 护理英语会话[M]. 北京：人民卫生出版社，2011.

[5] 曹红. 护理英语[M]. 北京：高等教育出版社，2005.

[6] 陈迎. 新职业英语医护英语[M]. 北京：外语教学与研究出版社，2009.

[7] 张燕，章国英. 医学英语视听说教程[M]. 北京：高等教育出版社，2008.

[8] 江晓东. 实用护理英语[M]. 重庆：重庆大学出版社，2008.

[9] 何萍. 医学基础英语[M]. 重庆：重庆大学出版社，2008.

[10] Jimmy Lin. 涉外护理英语情景对话[M]. 北京：外语教学与研究出版社，2006.

[11] 李敏. 专业英语[M]. 北京：高等教育出版社，2005.

[12] 王凯，刘兰兰. 医学英语会话[M]. 北京：化学工业出版社，2009.